HERBAL PLEASURES

HERBAL PLEASURES

FRANCES BALL

TYNRON PRESS
SCOTLAND

© Frances Ball, 1991

First published in 1991 by
Tynron Press
Stenhouse
Thornhill
Dumfriesshire DG3 4LD
Scotland

ISBN 1-85646-013-4

Cover illustration by Hazel McIntosh
Printed in Singapore by General Printing Services Pte Ltd

Contents

Colour Plates

Introduction

When I planted a small herb garden in the sixties, I had no idea that it marked the start of an interest that would continue for so many years. Sometimes in the town, sometimes in the country, I have planted and used changing groups of herbs. During those same years, more herbs have become available, and more people have discovered the pleasures of a growing range of plants.

I share my pastime with my husband, Larry, who has taken the photographs for this book. We have visited country fairs, gardens and parks — and searched for elusive wild herbs. We have tried products, remedies and recipes. His knowledge of the countryside and gardens has been a great help to me — also his comments on everything we have tried and tested. Our interest in herbs has grown as we worked on this book.

Frances Ball
1990

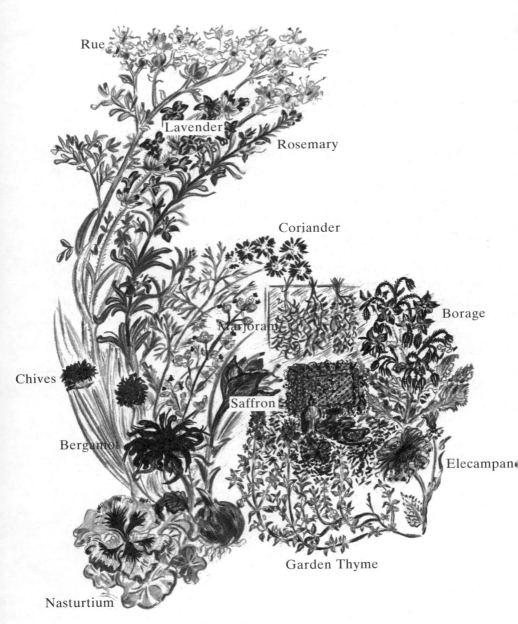

Rue

Lavender

Rosemary

Coriander

Marjoram

Borage

Chives

Saffron

Bergamot

Elecampane

Garden Thyme

Nasturtium

The twelve herbs illustrated on the cover.

Fact and Fancy

Herbs have been one of life's pleasures for many centuries. They were also one of life's necessities when 'green medicine' was the only kind available, and when meat needed a strong sauce to disguise its unrefrigerated age. From those years come the traditions that surround the most valued herbs — some factual and some fanciful — but all of them beguiling. Whether you accept them or not, they can add to the pleasure of using any herb, and provide a link across the centuries to the work of the early herbalists and the ancient green magic of plant lore.

After a period of neglect, herbs have become popular once again. Eating habits have again changed, more people have become interested in gardening, and alternative medicine has challenged many 'modern' ideas. Herbs have gained ground, and a wide variety of plants and products are now available. Generally this is good news, but sometimes the images surrounding herbs are exploited by advertisers or designers. A few of the products labelled 'herbal' need careful examination.

It is easy to see why herbal connections can be so tempting. Past references to herbs have often proved potent. Few people use rue today (though they could) but many would recognise it as the herb from Ophelia's sad speech: '. . . there's rue for you; and here's some for me: — we may call it herb-grace o' Sundays: — O, you must wear your rue with a difference. . .' Such memorable images surround many herbs.

The use of herbs to evoke the spirit of special places has given them further strong associations. And it is not only adults who encounter these. Many children have become aware of an idyllic countryside where real and imagined past are merged — a land of hillsides and hedgerows where the scent of thyme lingers in the morning air, and the rabbits disappear beneath a carpet of herbs. In *The Hobbit*, Tolkien shows us Bilbo Baggins in just such a place:

1

He nibbled a bit of sorrel, and he drank from a small mountain-stream that crossed the path, and he ate three wild strawberries he found on its bank, but it was not much food.

They still went on and on. The rough path disappeared. The bushes, and the long grasses between the boulders, the patches of rabbit-cropped turf, the thyme and the sage and the marjoram, and the yellow rockroses all vanished . . .

Like this distant scene, many of our local plants have also vanished — not just from view but from the highways and byways where they were once gathered. Today, you must search a little further for the wild herbs which many herbalists claim are more potent than their cultivated relatives. But they can still be found.

In a technological age, herbs provide a natural pleasure: a scent, or taste, or cure that has lost none of its charm over the years. And modern research has validated the traditional uses of many herbs.

Throughout this book, emphasis is placed on the value of herbs to enhance such pleasures as eating, drinking, sending gifts or relaxing in the garden on a warm evening. The remaining pages of this chapter give details of fifteen popular herbs. You will find information about their growth and uses, followed by some of the images and traditions associated with them.

Chives   *Allium schoenoprasum*

Height   about 12 cms   *Part used*   leaves

Cultivation

Grows from seed or root division. Native to northern Europe but now rarely seen wild except on a few limestone cliffs and riverbanks. There is also a larger, stronger variety called Chinese Chives (*Allium tuberosum*).

Uses

Culinary — its mild onion flavour makes it particularly suitable for use as a garnish on such things as salads, cream cheese and eggs.

Medicinal — not used medically though other members of the onion family, particularly garlic, have various uses.

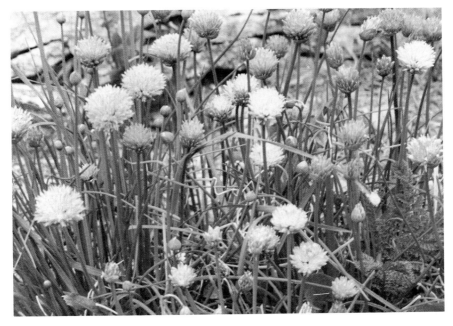

Chives

Images and associations

Although well-established for culinary use, chives have otherwise been given little attention by herbalists.

In the seventeenth century, Culpeper wrote: 'I confess I had not added these had it not been for a country gentleman, who by a letter certified to me that amongst herbs I had left these out'. He refers to them as chives or 'cives'.

Comfrey *Symphytum officinale*

Height   about 1 metre   *Parts used*   roots and leaves

Cultivation

Can be grown from seed or by root division and root cutting. It has quite deep roots and prefers a rich soil. A damp site is best and some watering may be required on dry soils.

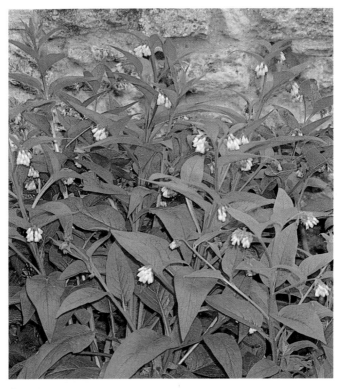

Comfrey

Uses

Culinary — the fresh leaves can be used as a vegetable or in salad. They can also be chopped and used in a white sauce as for parsley.

Medicinal — comfrey has long been used for medicinal purposes. The leaves and root can be applied as a poultice to wounds. The root is used in the treatment of internal ulcers and diarrhoea.

Other uses — the dried leaves can be used as a substitute for tea.

Note — excessive use of comfrey is not recommended as some recent studies have suggested that it may have some side-effects.

Images and associations

Known to the Greeks and Romans, and mentioned by Dioscorides as a medicinal herb.

Used during medieval times to treat battle wounds. This gave rise to its old names of 'knitbone' and 'boneset'. The Saracens used it for this purpose during the Crusades.

Used as a healing herb in many cultures including that of the gypsies.

The most common cultivated variety is Russian comfrey (*Symphytum peregrinum*). This was introduced into Britain by Henry Doubleday in the nineteenth century. The research association which bears his name continues his work with comfrey and is now well-known for its work on organic crops and cultivation. Comfrey is often used as an organic compost.

Dill *Anethum graveolens*

Height up to about 1 metre   *Parts used* leaves and seeds

Cultivation

An annual which will usually grow easily from seed. Likes quite a rich moist soil. It will self-seed if allowed to flower. Its delicate leaves are similar in appearance to fennel.

Uses

Culinary — popular as a flavouring for pickled cucumbers. Used in Scandinavian dishes such as gravad lax, and in sour cream sauces. The seeds are also added to some cakes and pastries.

Medicinal — long used to make dill water which helps ease children to sleep. Also good for digestive problems.

Other uses — the seeds are sometimes chewed to freshen the breath.

Images and associations

Its popular name dill probably comes from the Norse word 'dilla' meaning to lull.

A bag of dill carried over the heart was said to ward off the evil eye — the power of some people to bewitch, injure or kill merely by a potent glance. However, dill was also believed to be an ingredient in some witches' potions.

It has long been grown in England, and was sufficiently common for Addison to write three centuries ago:

> I am always pleased with that time of year when it is proper for the picking of dill and cucumbers.

Fennel *Foeniculum vulgare*

Height   about 1½ metres

Parts used   leaves, stems, seeds and roots

Fennel

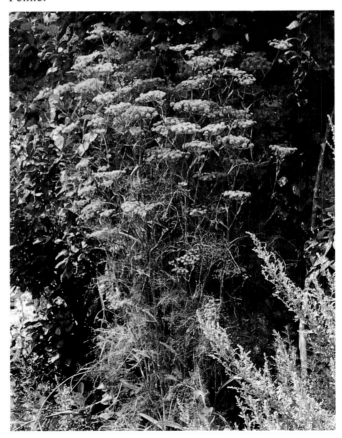

Cultivation

A biennial or perennial which grows easily in a sunny, sheltered position. Can be grown from seed or root division. Dislikes clay but otherwise quite tolerant.

Uses

Culinary — its classic use is with fish. The leaves or stems are used as a garnish or added to a sauce. Sometimes used with chicken or pork. The seeds can be added to apple pies, and in Italy they are scattered on bread and rolls. If the stems are to be eaten, Florence Fennel (*Finnocchio*) is the best variety to use. They are the most usual ingredient in fennel sauce with fish. The root can also be eaten as a vegetable.

Medicinal — fennel tea may be taken for indigestion.

Other uses — the seeds are sometimes chewed as a breath freshener.

Images and associations

The Greeks considered fennel to be an aid to slenderness. It has also long been regarded as an aphrodisiac, rejuvenator and fortifier.

The poor of the seventeenth century used to drink fennel tea to allay the pangs of hunger.

Chaucer wrote of it:

> Downe by a little path I fond
> Of mintes full and fennell greene.

It is also mentioned in Longfellow's *The Goblet of Life*:

> Above the lowly plant it towers,
> The fennel with its yellow flowers,
> And, in an earlier age than ours,
> Was gifted with wondrous powers,
> Lost vision to restore.

It is used in many areas of Europe, and is, for example, mentioned by the Russian writer Isaac Babel: 'A comparison must be. . . as natural as the smell of fennel.'

Feverfew *Tanacetum parthenium*

(sometimes also called *Chrysanthemum parthenium*)

Height   about 80 cms   *Part used*   leaves

Cultivation

A perennial which can be grown from seed, cutting or root division. Its appearance makes it suitable in a herb or cottage garden, and once established it usually grows well.

Uses

Culinary — although it is not regarded as a culinary herb, those taking it medicinally sometimes add a leaf or two to salads and sandwiches. Others find the fresh leaves can cause blisters in the mouth.

Medicinal — most often used by those suffering from migraine or

Feverfew

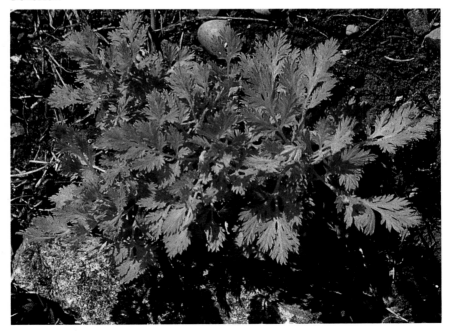

arthritis. Clinical trials in the late seventies supported the use of feverfew for migraine though some side-effects can occur.

Other uses — sometimes used in insecticides.

Images and associations

Its common name feverfew comes from its traditional use against fever.

Used by the Romans as a cure for headache, possibly also for hangover.

Also known to the Greeks. Plutarch describes its use to help a workman injured when he fell from the Parthenon.

The bright yellow and white flowers are a distinctive feature of the plant, probably giving rise to its nickname of 'bachelor's buttons'.

Traditionally, this has been a herb used by women. Culpeper recommended its use in wine, sometimes with the addition of mace or nutmeg, to help menstruation or to relieve problems following childbirth.

French Tarragon *Artemisia dracunculus*

Height   about 80 cms   *Part used*   leaves

Cultivation

A perennial which grows most easily from cuttings or root division. A sheltered, sunny site is required. This is a variable plant which must be chosen with care. If you have a friend with a well-flavoured example, try to obtain a cutting. French tarragon has a much more delicate flavour than Russian tarragon.

Uses

Culinary — can be used to make your own version of fines herbes with equal proportions of chervil, parsley and chives. A subtle herb most often used with such things as eggs, chicken and fish. Also used to make tarragon vinegar.

Medicinal — rarely used as a medicinal herb today though its inclusion in food is considered good for digestion. Once considered a cure for toothache.

Other uses — as a flavouring in some liqueurs.

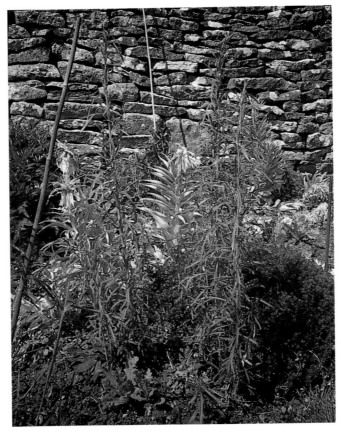

French Tarragon

Images and associations

Its name means 'little dragon' and probably refers to its coiled roots.

The Greeks believed that the *artemisia* group of plants (which includes southernwood and wormwood) was discovered by the goddess Diana.

Perhaps because it is mainly a culinary herb, fewer traditions have become associated with tarragon than with other popular herbs. It is known chiefly through its use in such classic dishes as poulet à l'estragon, sauce bearnaise, and sauce tartare.

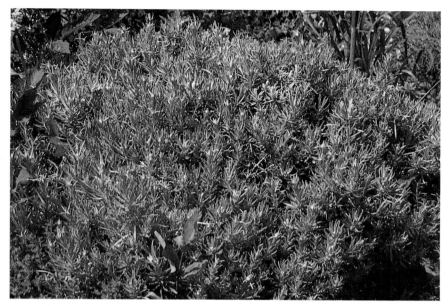

Lavender

Lavender *Lavandula officinalis*

Height   about 60 cms   *Parts used*   flowers and leaves

Cultivation

A perennial which can be grown from seed or cuttings. Prefers a light soil and sunny position. A popular garden plant which usually grows easily.

Uses

Culinary — occasionally used in conserves. Also used with light meats such as rabbit. The dried flower heads are tied in muslin as for bouquet garni, and removed before serving.

Medicinal — good for burns and stings. A relaxing herb with sedative properties. Inhalations recommended for coughs. The oil is widely used in aromatherapy.

Other uses — best known for its use in perfumes and scented sachets.

Images and associations

English lavender water has been popular and quite widely available since the eighteenth century.

It is a herb particularly associated with London. There were once extensive lavender fields at Mitcham, now remembered in local names such as Lavender Road.

The film, *The Lavender Hill Mob*, produced by Ealing Studios, immortalises another area of London known for its lavender. The side streets are: Lavender Gardens, Lavender Walk, and Lavender Sweep.

Street cries such as 'Come buy! Come buy my sweet lavender!' were common in Victorian London. Their distinctive cries have been used in musicals like Lionel Bart's *Oliver!* to evoke the feeling of the period.

Lavender is known to many children through the nursery rhyme:

Lavender's blue, dilly, dilly, lavender's green,
When I am king, dilly, dilly, you will be queen.

Mint *Mentha spicata*

Height   25-100 cms   *Part used*   leaves

Cultivation

A perennial best grown from cuttings — it rarely grows from seed. Its aroma may also deteriorate if it is left unmoved for too long on the same site.

Uses

Culinary — widely used in mint sauce with lamb. It is also used with many cold dishes — both salad and fruit. Mint jelly made with apples or plums illustrates its use as a delicate flavouring, while its use in 'bullseyes' shows its strength.

Medicinal — often used against catarrh or the common cold, where the herbal aroma or oil is inhaled. Also used in massage oils and liniments.

Other uses — various cosmetic and dental uses. Also used in some liqueurs.

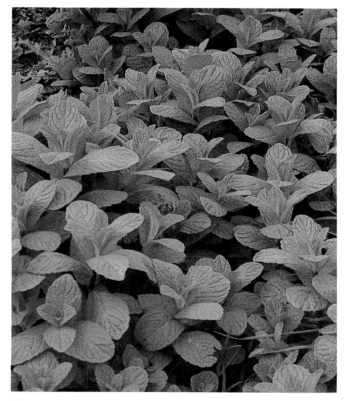

Mint

Images and associations

Long used around the shores of the Mediterranean where there are many legends about its origins. One such story tells how Pluto was attracted to the nymph *Mentha*. Persephone, his jealous wife, trod her underfoot and Pluto was unable to save her. All he could do was change her into a fragrant herb which remained sacred to him.

One of Ovid's tales refers to mint as a symbol of hospitality, and Pliny regarded it as a useful medicinal herb.

The Roman legions carried mint to most parts of the Empire and during the Middle Ages it was usually found in monastery gardens, among other herbs.

Gives its distinctive flavour to the classic drink, 'Mint Julep'.

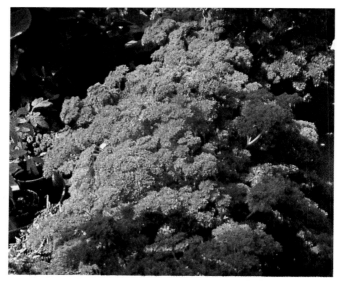

Parsley

Parsley *Petroselinum crispum*

Height   about 30 cms

Parts used   roots, leaves and seeds

Cultivation

Can be difficult to grow from seed. The seeds are often slow to germinate. Should not be sown too deep — a covering of 1 cm is sufficient. It is a hardy biennial which will normally go to seed the spring after sowing.

Uses

Culinary — best known for its use in parsley sauce or bouquet garni, and as a fresh garnish.

Medicinal — a rich source of vitamin C, particularly if used fresh. Recommended for treating urinary infections.

Other uses — long used as a breath freshener, particularly as an antidote to garlic. Oil from the fresh seeds is used for medicines and as a flavouring for liqueurs.

Images and associations

Used by the Greeks as a decoration at funerals. Hercules was said to have worn a garland of parsley.

During the Middle Ages it was believed that you could kill your enemy if you shouted his/her name while pulling a root of parsley.

Said to be slow to germinate because it goes to the devil and back several times before it comes up.

Believed to flourish where the 'missus' is master.

Said to bring happiness and good fortune if sown on Good Friday.

Claimed to cure sick fish if thrown into the water.

More recently mentioned by Simon and Garfunkel in *Scarborough Fair*:

Are you going to Scarborough Fair?
Parsley, sage, rosemary and thyme,
Remember me to one who is there,
She once was a true love of mine.

Rosemary *Rosmarinus officinalis*

Height   about 180 cms   *Parts used*   leaves and wood

Cultivation

Choose a sheltered, sunny spot and grow from seed, or from cuttings of non-flowering shoots. It can be grown as an individual plant or as a hedge. If grown as a hedge, a supply of sprigs is assured whenever it is trimmed.

Uses

Culinary — most often used with lamb or game, but also good with pork or poultry. It is a strongly flavoured herb which should be removed from food before serving.

Medicinal — an infusion (see page 88) can be taken to relieve headaches or to aid the circulation.

Other uses — an infusion can be used as a hair rinse, particularly for dark hair. And an infusion with borax (sodium pyroborate) gets rid of dandruff. Sprigs of rosemary produce a pleasant incense when burned. The wood was used to make lutes and carpenters' rules.

Images and associations

Long recognised for its medicinal properties, it is mentioned in Cervantes' *Don Quixote*:

'Sir, whoever you are, be so very kind as to give us a little rosemary, some oil, some salt, and some wine, for they are needed to heal one of the best knights errant in the world. . .'

It was a favourite herb in Tudor times, when Sir Thomas More wrote that:

As for rosemarie I lette it runne all over my garden walls, not onlie because my bees love it, but because it is the herb sacred to remembrance and to friendship, whence a sprig of it hath a dumb language.

Rosemary

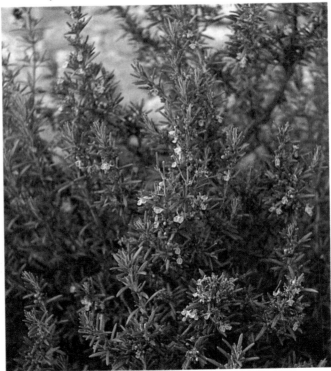

Often used in ceremonies, particularly weddings. For example, Anne of Cleves took a wreath of rosemary to the altar when she married Henry VIII.

It was one of the chief ingredients of Hungary Water, the famous perfumed water made since the fourteenth century. Charles Perrault describes how Hungary Water was used to massage the temples of 'Sleeping Beauty' when she had pricked her finger.

Rue . *Ruta graveolens*

Height   about 50 cms   *Part used*   leaves

Cultivation

Can be grown from seeds or cuttings during spring. It can also be grown from root division but this requires care. A perennial which likes a well-drained soil and a sheltered, sunny position.

Uses

Culinary — the leaves are occasionally used to give a peppery flavour to salads.

Medicinal — long valued for its medicinal properties in European and Chinese herbal medicine. Today, it is chiefly known for its use in treating headaches and eyestrain.

Other uses — it was used in the making of 'sack', a traditional wine from Spain and the Canaries. The oil is used in the making of perfumes.

Images and associations

Often called 'Herb of Grace' and known by this name from Ophelia's speech in Hamlet.

Used as a symbol of regret and repentance, and for this reason it was traditionally carried by judges at the assizes. It was also believed to help prevent gaol fever, and is referred to in this context by Dickens in *A Tale of Two Cities*.

It was one ingredient of the poison antidotes used by Mithridates, and was mentioned by Aristotle for its use as an aid to digestion.

Also one of the herbs included in plague antidotes during the

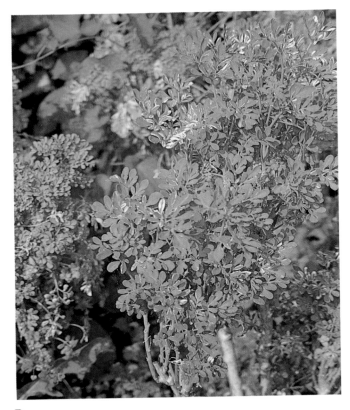

Rue

Middle Ages. Recommended by Culpeper during the seventeenth century when used with dill: 'A decoction made with dried dill leaves eases all inward pains and torments'.

Sage *Salvia officinalis*

Height   about 45 cms   *Part used*   leaves

Cultivation

A perennial best grown from cuttings. It prefers a sheltered, warm site but will tolerate a little shade. To maintain its aroma, it can be divided or moved every two to three years.

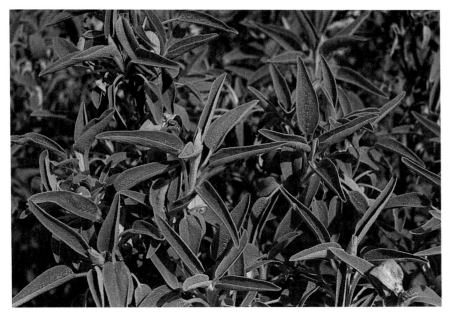

Sage
Uses

Culinary — one of the most popular herbs — frequently used in sage and onion stuffing. Sometimes used with pasta. It should be used sparingly as its strong flavour can overwhelm other herbs or food with a delicate flavour. Also used in sage cheese, and occasionally as a flavouring in bread.

Medicinal — long recommended as a healing herb. Used in mouthwashes and gargles for protection against sore throats. Sage 'tobacco' is sometimes recommended for asthma sufferers.

Other uses — as a bee plant.

Images and associations

The sacred herb of Zeus for the Greeks, and Jupiter for the Romans.

Always highly regarded as a healing herb — its name 'salvia' coming from 'salvare', the Latin word for save. It was given to women to help them conceive, and used for protection during times of plague.

Sage tea has been highly regarded for many centuries. The Chinese used to trade large quantities of their tea with the Dutch in return for sage tea.

Sage is not native to Britain but has been grown locally for many years. In the sixteenth century, Gerard noted that sage could be found in many parts of London '. . . especially in the fields of Holborne neare unto Graye's Inn, on the highway by the end of a brickewall.'

In England, one tradition was that with sage sprigs girls could envisage their future husbands on Midsummer' Eve just after sunset. At night, the boy would appear to sprinkle rose-water on the smock of his future wife.

Sweet Basil *Ocimum basilicum*

Height   about 45 cms   *Parts used*   leaves and roots

Cultivation

Sweet basil is not easily grown outdoors from seed in this country where it is regarded as a semi-hardy annual. Occasionally, it will survive in a very sheltered garden. You could grow it indoors, or use it in a pot suitable for moving indoors and outdoors according to the weather.

Uses

Culinary — best known for its use in tomato and pasta dishes. It can be used very simply, for example, chopped and added to French dressing — then poured over fresh, sliced tomatoes.

Medicinal — a standard infusion (see page 88) is considered beneficial for stomach troubles.

Other uses — it is sometimes planted as an insect repellant and is used with tomatoes in 'companion planting'. In its native India, where the plant is a perennial, the roots are sometimes carved into beads.

Images and associations

In India, where it is known as 'tulasi', basil is the sacred herb of the Hindu gods, Krishna and Vishnu.

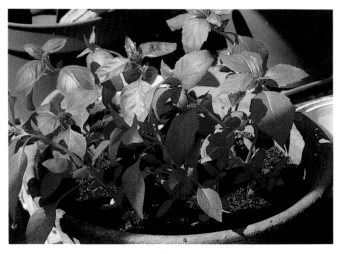

Sweet Basil

In Europe, the Greeks regarded it highly. It was said that only the sovereign could cut it and only with a golden sickle. Its name *basilicum* may have come from the Greek word for kingly or royal.

In Italy it was seen as a symbol of love. Similarly, in Romania, the tradition was that a boy accepting a sprig of basil from his girl had become engaged.

In Britain, it is known through Keats' poem 'Isabella and The Pot of Basil'.

One tradition is that St. Helena found the herb beneath the cross.

The herbalist, Gerard, commented that it '. . . cureth the infirmities of the heart, (and) taketh away sorrowfulness which cometh of melancholia and maketh a man merry and glad.'

Sweet Marjoram *Origanum majorana*

Height about 30 cms   *Part used* leaves

Cultivation

A perennial which likes a well-drained, sunny site. It can be grown from root division, or from seeds which can be sown outdoors in June.

Uses

Culinary — one of the herbs included in bouquet garni. Widely used in savoury meat and vegetable dishes. Also popular as a flavouring for sausages.

Medicinal — an infusion (see page 88) will help ease insomnia. It also aids digestion. Marjoram oil is sometimes used externally for rheumatic pains.

Other uses — sometimes used to provide the bitter flavour in beer, particularly when hops were not available. An infusion used as a hair rinse is suitable for all hair types.

Images and associations

Wild marjoram (*Origanum vulgare*) is found in many areas, and is mentioned by Richard Adams in *Watership Down*: 'The air was heavy with thick, herbal smells, as though it were already late June; the water-mint and marjoram, not yet flowering, gave off scent from their leaves and here and there an early meadow-sweet stood in bloom.'

Golden Marjoram

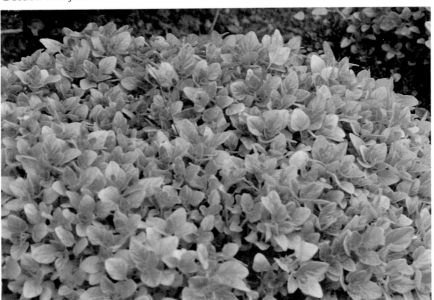

It also occurs in Blackmore's *Lorna Doone*: 'I assure them I am good inside, and not a bit of rue in me; only queer knots as of marjoram. . .'

The Greeks and Romans planted it on graves, and in the Middle Ages it was sometimes used as a charm against witchcraft.

Like many herbs, it occurs in the Bible: 'Moses summoned all the elders of Israel and said to them, 'Go at once and get sheep for your families and slaughter the Passover. Then take a bunch of marjoram, dip it in the blood in the basin and smear some blood from the basin on the lintel and the two door posts'.

Thyme *Thymus vulgaris*

Height   about 30 cms   *Part used*   leaves

Cultivation

Although thyme can be grown from seed, it is more easily grown from cuttings taken in early summer. Roots can also be divided in autumn. It is a perennial which likes a well-drained soil and a sheltered position.

Thyme

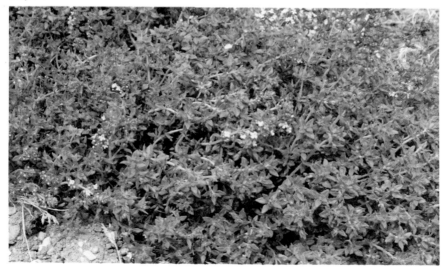

Uses

Culinary — one of the herbs used in bouquet garni — also used alone in many savoury dishes. Lemon thyme (*Thymus citriodorus*) is similar in appearance but has a pleasant lemon fragrance which enhances fruit dishes. It is also used with fish and veal.

Medicinal — an infusion (see page 88) of thyme is useful as a gargle to ease sore throats. The oil from the plant has traditionally been used against hookworm.

Other uses — in hair rinses and various cosmetic preparations.

Images and associations

In Shakespeare's *A Midsummer Night's Dream*, Oberon seeks Titania on 'a bank where the wild thyme blows'.

Legend has always associated wild thyme (*Thymus serpyllum*) with fairies, and in *A Garden of Herbs*, E.S. Rohde gives an old recipe '. . . to enable one to see the Fairies'. The thyme must be gathered from the east near a fairy throne and the '. . . vial glasses in which the liquid is made must first be washed with rose-water and marygolde water'.

Kipling, in his poem *Sussex*, describes wild thyme smelling 'like dawn in paradise'.

Thyme appears alongside other herbs in Tolkien's *The Lord of the Rings*:

South and west it looked towards the warm lower vales of Anduin, shielded from the east by the Ephel Duath and not yet under the mountain shadow. . . Many great trees grew there, planted long ago, falling into untended age amid a riot of careless descendants; and groves and thickets there were of tamarisk and terebinth, of olive and of bay: and there were juniper and myrtles; and thymes that grew in bushes, or with woody creeping stems mantled in deep tapestries the hidden stones. . .

A Taste of Herbs

Food prepared with herbs can provide a wide range of flavours and effects. You may want the light, subtle flavours of *nouvelle cuisine* — or the warm, exciting taste of Jhal farzi cooked with your own blend of herbs and spices. This versatility is one of the attractions of herbs.

Many herbs also have meanings, or convey messages, that can give a meal particular significance. This advantage can be used on any scale from public functions to intimate private dinners. Some traditional meals of this type have continued for many years. The central feature of the long-established *Boar's Head Ceremony* at Queen's College, Oxford, is the cooked and glazed boar's head decorated with holly, mistletoe, bay and rosemary. Those assembled sing the *Boar's Head Carol* which includes the lines:

The Boar's Head in hand bear I,
Bedeck'd with bays and rosemary. . .

They are then presented with sprigs of rosemary with all its associations of remembrance and friendship.

Using herbs in this way can add to the pleasure of special meals at home. There are many herbs associated with love or affection that would enhance an anniversary meal for two, the return or departure of friends, and similar occasions. Basil is one herb well-suited to this use. A meal garnished or flavoured with basil could be accompanied by a card decorated with a sprig of basil, and a gift.

Other images surrounding herbs come from the places in which they are found: from open hillsides to formal gardens. You may want to select a recipe from any point along this spectrum. Perhaps you are planning a special picnic to be eaten beside a favourite stream or view. It could include some fresh, wild herbs. The late summer months are good for picking wild thyme and marjoram. The freshness and simplicity of wild herbs are captured by John Clare in

25

The Shepherd's Calendar:

> The brook resumes her summer dresses,
> Purling 'neath grass and water-cresses,
> And mint and flagleaf, swording high
> Their blooms to the unheeding eye. . .

Unspoilt countryside, seen by few, with its plants reflected in a glittering stream, could provide a whole range of images for cool green salads and refreshing mint juleps.

This same countryside, loved by many but lived in by few, has always served many purposes — not least to supply produce for a very different style of country life. This is the life mockingly celebrated, but also greatly enjoyed, by Lord Byron:

> Lord Henry and his Lady were the hosts;
> The party we have touched on were the guests.
> Their table was a board to tempt even ghosts
> To pass the Styx for more substantial feasts.
> I will not dwell upon ragouts or roasts,
> Albeit all human history attests
> That happiness for man — the hungry sinner! —
> Since Eve ate apples, much depends on dinner.

Possibly because many well-known herb gardens are in the grounds of large country houses, herbs are often associated with this type of lifestyle. There is some truth in this — and it is the source of some magnificent herb recipes — but it does obscure the wide use of herbs in many lifestyles and a wide range of recipes.

Your own use of herbs might include many styles, probably your own collection of personal recipes. If you are experimenting, or if you are developing your own selection of fresh and dried herbs, there are several things to keep in mind:

Fresh or dried?

Even if you grow fresh herbs, and have a greenhouse for those herbs not usually available in winter, you are likely to need some dried herbs. Recipes do not always specify whether the herbs they include are fresh or dried but if they do, and you are substituting one for the other, it should be kept in mind that one ounce of dried herbs is roughly equivalent to three ounces of fresh herbs. In most cases, the fresh herb is preferable to the dried but some herbs such as lovage, marjoram, sage and savory do dry quite well. Annuals such as chives and basil do not usually dry well as their essential oils are too volatile. If you need to store some, they will last about six months if frozen.

When shortages occur, it is now possible to buy dried *and* fresh herbs at most good supermarkets. These can be used alongside those you have grown or collected.

Collecting wild or cultivated herbs

If you require only a small sprig or a few leaves, they can be picked whenever they are available. In the case of wild herbs, this is all that should be picked. The remainder of the plant should be left to continue growing.

When larger amounts are required, or a herb is being collected for annual drying, some preparation will be necessary. Herb leaves will be at their best for drying just before their flowers are in full bloom. They should also be picked when they are dry and insect-free.

If the plant is being grown for its flowers, they should be cut when fully open. For culinary use, these flowers might include roses, nasturtiums, violets or marigolds.

If the seeds are required — dill, fennel or coriander, for example — cut or pull up the whole plant. It can then be hung above sheets of paper while the seeds fall.

Plants collected for their roots (dandelion or horseradish, for example) are best removed in autumn, and carefully cleaned.

Drying

For ordinary domestic use, most herbs can be dried in bunches in any room or shed which is airy and *not* damp. Herbs will not usually dry well in a kitchen — but an airing cupboard, dry loft or empty wardrobe could be suitable. It is best to tie only a few sprigs together so that all the leaves dry well. I used to dry mine on muslin racks in a cupboard gently heated by warm pipes. The space was shared by various household items but worked well for herbs.

Storing

When the herbs are completely dry, pick off the leaves and store whole, or in pieces. If small pieces are preferred, use a coffee grinder. Store in an airtight container in a dark place. If you want to store your herbs on shelves in the kitchen, for example, use containers which do not let in the light.

If a herb is available that you do not usually use, it is always best to store some. Dried herbs last for some time. The most likely cause of problems with dried herbs is moisture. Check your supply of dried herbs regularly to make sure that none of them are becoming damp or mouldy. Some herbs, such as parsley, do not look particularly attractive when dried. This is not a problem if they provide enough flavour but they would not be useful as a garnish.

The remaining pages of this chapter set out a selection of recipes which can easily be tried out at home. There are seasonal herb recipes, classic herb recipes, and some recipes for children.

Four Seasonal Herb Recipes

Spring

Roast Lamb with Rosemary

Items required

roasting lamb
cooking oil

rosemary — several sprigs
salt and pepper

Preparation

1. About one hour before you put the lamb into the oven, finely chop half the sprigs of rosemary.
2. Mix these with two tablespoons of cooking oil seasoned with salt and pepper.
3. Rub the mixture over the lamb, then slice the skin in a few places and insert the ends of the uncut sprigs. Leave in a cool place.
4. One hour later, put the meat into an oven pre-heated to 220° C/425° F for about ten minutes. Then reduce to 180° C/350° F until ready.

5. Serve with new potatoes and peas.

Summer

Egg Mayonnaise with Nasturtium Leaves and Paprika

Items required

Six hard-boiled eggs
About ten nasturtium leaves
Paprika to garnish

For the mayonnaise:
  2 egg yolks
  pepper and salt to taste
  ½ teaspoon paprika
  ½ pint good oil
  2 tablespoons vinegar
  1 tablespoon lemon juice

Preparation

Using a beater or blender:
1. Put egg yolks, salt, pepper and paprika into a bowl and mix thoroughly.
2. Start adding the oil drop by drop while mixing.
3. When about a quarter of the oil has been added, start adding the mixed vinegar and lemon alternately with the oil — also drop by drop.
4. Continue mixing until all the ingredients have been added and the mayonnaise has thickened.

Then:
Arrange the nasturtium leaves to form a bed for the boiled eggs. Place the eggs on the leaves and pour mayonnaise over them. Sprinkle with paprika.

Autumn

Silver Leaf Apple Jelly

Items required

Cooking apples
Sugar (two pounds for each two pints of the strained liquid obtained from the apples)

Bouquet of 'silver leaf' herbs:

1 lavender head
1 sprig lemon thyme   for each two pints of the strained
1 sprig pineapple sage   liquid
A jelly bag

Preparation

1. Cut the apples but do not peel or core them. Add ½ pint of water for each pound of fruit.
2. Bring the cut apples and water to the boil, then simmer until pulped.
3. Put the pulp through a jelly bag and leave to strain for several hours.
4. Measure the juice. For each two pints of juice, add two pounds of sugar and one 'silver leaf' bouquet.
5. Stir the mixture.
6. Boil rapidly until set — without stirring. This will take about 5-10 minutes.
7. Test for setting by removing the jelly from the heat, putting a spoonful on a saucer and leaving to cool. The jelly is ready when this sample forms a skin or wrinkles when moved with the spoon.
8. Remove any scum from the surface of the jelly and pour into warm jars.
9. Fill the jars as near to the top as possible. Add wax circles, and cling film or something similar, and store until required.

Winter

Chicken Soup with Tarragon Dumplings

Items required

Chicken soup:
1 chicken carcass
8-10 ozs cooked chicken
2 tablespoons cooking oil
3 ozs plain flour

salt and pepper
a sprig of tarragon
2 onions

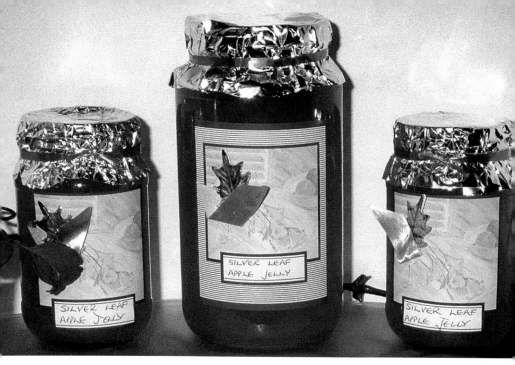

△ Silver Leaf apple jelly.

▽ Cards decorated with herbs.

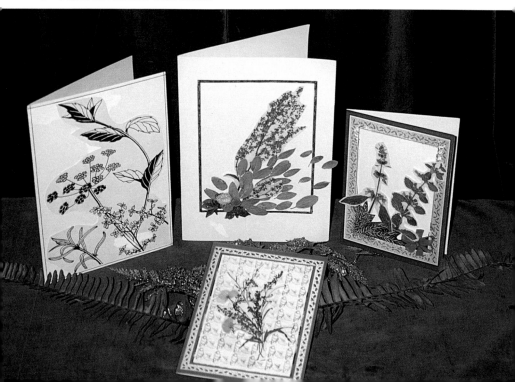

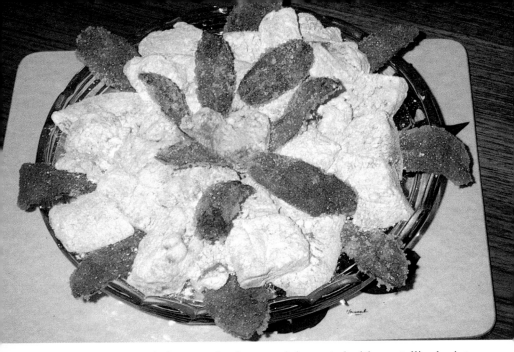

△ Mint treats, made in several colours and decorated with crystallised mint leaves.

▽ Omelette with fines herbes.

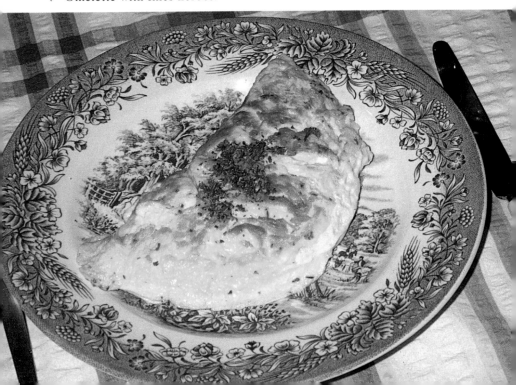

Tarragon dumplings:

4 ozs self raising flour   2 teaspoons finely chopped
2 ozs shredded suet (e.g. Atora)   tarragon
salt and pepper

Preparation

1. Simmer the chicken carcass for at least half an hour then strain off the stock.
2. Fry the onions in the oil until soft, then stir in the flour.
3. Add the stock slowly, gradually bringing the mixed liquid to the boil.
4. Add the meat and seasoning, then simmer for a few more minutes.
5. Use a blender to puree the soup, then store or reheat as required for use with the dumplings.

Dumplings

1. Mix all the ingredients together and add enough cold water to form a dough.
2. Separate into tiny balls and drop into the soup to cook.

Four Classic Herb Recipes

Bouquet Garni

This is probably the best-known of the classic French herb mixtures, particularly for stocks, soups and stews. The usual ingredients are: one part bay, one part thyme and three parts parsley. Variations often include marjoram, or fennel if a fish dish is being prepared. The herbs are wrapped in muslin during preparation of the meal, and removed when it is ready.

Beef and Root Casserole with Bouquet Garni

Items required

1½ lbs stewing steak cut into   ½ cup stock
   small pieces   ½ cup white wine

1 onion	bouquet garni
1 carrot	2 ozs flour
1 small turnip	cooking oil
½ medium swede	salt and pepper

Preparation

1. Gently fry the onion in the cooking oil.
2. Roll the cut pieces of meat in the flour, salt and pepper.
3. Brown the meat in the oil with the onions.
4. Blend in the wine and stock — bring it to the boil, and cook until it thickens.
5. Add the vegetables — chopped quite small — and the bouquet garni.
6. Cover and cook at 350° F/180° C for about 2 hours.
7. Remove the bouquet garni when ready.
8. Serve with dumplings or boiled potatoes.

Fines Herbes

Like bouquet garni, this is a classic French herb mixture which remains basically unchanged but may have minor variations to suit personal taste. Usually, it is a mixture of equal parts of parsley, chives, chervil and tarragon. If you grow your own herbs, you can use the mixture fresh when all the herbs are available. You may also want to keep some of the mixture for use when fresh herbs are not available. This is not a mixture of herbs that dries particularly well so some could be stored frozen if you have space available.

The fines herbes mixture is most often used in egg dishes, with white fish or light meats.

Omelette with Fines Herbes

Items required

4 eggs	salt and pepper
2 ozs butter	fines herbes

Preparation

1. Start heating the butter in a heavy frying pan.

2. Break the eggs into a basin with salt and pepper, and some of the fines herbes.
3. Beat the egg mixture until the yolks and whites are just blended.
4. When the butter foams but has not changed colour, pour the mixture into the pan.
5. As it starts to set, lift the edges to allow any uncooked mixture to run underneath.
6. When lightly set on top, fold in half, garnish with some more fines herbes, and serve at once.

Fish with Fennel

Fish with fennel is a classic combination used in many ways. These include red mullet garnished with fennel, fish and salad with grated fennel root, and fish with fennel sauce. The following sauce is good with trout or mackerel.

Fennel Sauce

Items required

4 ozs chopped Florence fennel   2 ozs cream
½ pint fish stock   salt and pepper

Preparation

1. Simmer the fennel in the stock for about 10 minutes.
2. Put the fennel and stock into a blender and purée.
3. Pour into a dish, then beat in the cream.

Crystallised Rose Petals

This is also suitable for violets, nasturtiums, geranium leaves and mint leaves. The best rose petals to use are large, dark red ones.

Items required

Rose petals   Greaseproof paper
One lightly beaten egg white   Pastry brush
Caster sugar

Preparation

1. Rinse the petals and shake dry.
2. Brush both sides with egg white.
3. Cover both sides of the petals with sugar and shake off any loose sugar.
4. Put the petals onto greaseproof paper.
5. Use when dry and crisp.

Four Recipes for Children

Peanut Stuffing

Ingredients

4 ozs finely chopped onions
2 ozs finely chopped
   mushrooms
2 tablespoons cooking oil

2 teaspoons chopped parsley
   and parsley to garnish
3 ozs smooth or crunchy peanut
   butter
4 ozs breadcrumbs

Preparation

1. Gently heat the oil and cook the onions until slightly brown.
2. Stir in the mushrooms and parsley.
3. Add the peanut butter and breadcrumbs, then mix all the ingredients thoroughly.
4. Use to stuff chicken or turkey — or roll into balls and cook on a greased tray.
5. If prepared in balls, cook in oven with the meat for the last 30-40 minutes, and garnish with parsley.

Tom's Cheese and Tomato Pizza

A simple pizza which includes one herb — marjoram. This enhances the flavour and stimulates the appetite.

Ingredients

Base
6 ozs self-raising flour
salt and pepper

½ oz butter or fat
water

Topping

Small can of tomato puree   4 ozs grated cheese
Finely chopped marjoram

Preparation

1. Rub the butter into the flour and seasoning.
2. Add the water until the dough is manageable, and spread into a pizza shape on an ungreased baking tray.
3. Mix the tomato purée and marjoram, and spread over the pizza.
4. Bake for 20 minutes at 220° C/425° F, then add the grated cheese and serve.

Matthew's Hot Dog Relish

Ingredients

2 tablespoons cooking oil   2 tablespoons vinegar
2 cloves garlic   2 tablespoons tomato purée
1 finely chopped onion   4 tablespoons chopped mixed
                                    pickle
3 tablespoons cornflour   small cup of stock
1 tablespoon brown sugar

Preparation

1. Fry the onions and garlic gently in the oil.
2. Stir in the cornflour.
3. Add the tomato purée.
4. Slowly add the stock.
5. Add the vinegar, brown sugar and pickle, and mix thoroughly.
6. Serve hot or cold.

Mint Treats

Ingredients

2 tablespoons powdered   1 lb icing sugar
   gelatine   oil of peppermint
½ pint very hot water   green colouring
2 tablespoons lemon juice

Preparation

1. Sprinkle the gelatine into half the water and stir.
2. Dissolve the icing sugar in the other half of the water.
3. Mix the two liquids together, bring to the boil, and simmer for 20 minutes.
4. Add the lemon juice, colouring, and a few drops of peppermint oil. Turn into a tin or bowl.

When set, cut into pieces and roll in icing sugar. These sweets go well with crystallised mint leaves. If required, see the recipe for rose petals on page 35.

A Draught of Herbs

Herbal teas, or tisanes, were in use long before coffee or Indian and Chinese teas became available. They were neglected for many years while the new drinks dominated the market but recently sales of the most popular herbal flavours have revived. Some of these are taken for medicinal purposes but most are bought for their pleasant taste and as safer replacements for tea and coffee.

Criticism of tea and coffee is not new. During the seventeenth century when coffee was introduced into Britain, a broadsheet in London claimed that women had turned against it because it was weakening their husbands! But coffee survived, and coffee-drinking became respectable. It was valued for its ability to ward off sleep, and though it emerged that it contained caffeine, little notice was taken until more people sought healthier eating and drinking habits.

Caffeine tolerance varies greatly from person to person but heavy users (12-15 cups a day) can become edgy and may suffer mild 'withdrawal' symptoms if they decide to stop suddenly. Traditional English tea also contains caffeine but it is the tannin content that really tarnishes its genteel 'tea-room' image. In excess, tannin reduces the assimilation of B vitamins, and this eventually affects the absorption of iron. But if you plan to change your tea-drinking habits, check carefully first. Some herbal teas such as sage also contain tannin! But the amounts are relatively small.

If you like to stock a whole range of teas and coffees, you can buy de-caffeinated tea and coffee and a range of herbal teas for different purposes or times of day. Just as you can buy Indian breakfast teas, so can you buy herbal blends such as Morning Starter and Evening Peace. Popular herbal flavours include: Camomile, Apple and Cinnamon, Rosehip and Hibiscus, and Peppermint. These teas do not taste like Indian or Chinese teas (which come from a species of camellia). Some people find that herbal teas are an acquired taste, others try quite a few flavours before finding the one they like best.

But, just as some people like Earl Grey and others enjoy Lapsang Souchong, so some people enjoy bergamot and others prefer elderflower.

Most herbal teas come in tea bags. They can be taken with or without milk, and with or without sweetening. Some people enjoy them with honey and lemon. If you take them without milk, they look attractive served in heatproof glasses with holders.

In addition to the teas available commercially, it is also possible to produce your own. You can select these according to personal taste, or for a specific purpose: camomile at night for restful sleep, lime flower for headache, peppermint for digestion or rosemary for tension, for example. When making your tea, two teaspoons of dried herbs are usually sufficient for each cup. Brew the tea in a pot kept solely for herbal teas and strain before drinking.

You could also experiment with blends for many teas on sale are in fact blends of several flavours.

Make a note of the contents and proportions so that when you find a favourite you can repeat it. The following herbs could be tried individually or as blends:

Leaves

blackcurrant, blackberry, lemon balm, peppermint, sage, raspberry, rosemary, thyme, periwinkle, marjoram, bergamot.

Petals and flowers

rose, marigold, lime, elder, woodruff (with the leaves), camomile (with the leaves).

Seeds and hips

fennel, celery, rose.

As an alternative to coffee, dandelion roots make a surprisingly similar product. Although autumn is the best time to collect the roots, they can be gathered at any time of the year. They need to be well cleaned, then wrapped in foil and roasted in the oven at quite a high temperature. They will then crumble to a powder which looks very similar to bought powdered coffee. Like coffee, dandelion root has a distinctive aroma, and a similar but not identical taste.

Chicory (*Cichorium intybus*) is also a good substitute for coffee. The roots can be roasted in the same way as those from dandelion. The powder from chicory or dandelion roots can be mixed with bought coffee to produce your own blend.

Summer Drinks

Mint julep

This is probably the best-known of all the summer drinks made with herbs. It is delightfully cool and refreshing.

Items required

whisky	castor sugar
soda	lemon slices
ice	tall glasses
freshly-cut mint	

Preparation

1. Frost the edges of the glasses. To do this, put a little water in one bowl and a little sugar in the other. Dip each glass into the water, then into the sugar. Frost the edges in this way to a depth of about half an inch.
2. Put a level teaspoonful of sugar into each glass.
3 Put a few mint leaves into each glass.
4 Add a dash of soda and about half a glass of ice.
5. Add the whisky (one measure).
6. Stir and add a slice of lemon.

Iced Vermouth

Vermouth is a classic herb-flavoured drink. The exact ingredients of commercially-prepared vermouths are a closely guarded secret but wormwood is usually the main one.

You can make your own vermouth using red or white wine and a selection of herbs. These might include rosemary, southernwood, fennel, bay, tansy, angelica, camomile, lemon balm, lemon verbena, cinnamon, coriander, nutmeg, mixed spice or ginger. Choose a selection with flavours you like. They should also be ones likely to blend well together. Add them to the wine, and leave for several weeks. Strain and bottle when ready.

Your vermouth can then be served simply with ice or as a long drink with tonic added. The ice cubes can be set with sprigs of some of the same herbs used for steeping.

Traditional lemonade

Items required

6 lemons
½ lb sugar
6 pints boiling water

Preparation

1. Thinly slice the lemons and put them into a large jug.
2. Add the sugar and the boiling water.
3. Leave to cool overnight.
4. Strain.
5. Serve with some ice cubes set with herbs — mint is pleasant with the lemonade.

Winter Drinks

Mulled wine

Items required

1 bottle of red wine
5 cloves
cinnamon

thinly peeled orange rind
2 teaspoons dark brown sugar

Preparation

1. Boil the cloves, cinnamon, orange and brown sugar in half a pint of water.
2. Add the wine and reheat but do not boil.

Norfolk Punch

This can be obtained from various large stores and major off-licences. It contains a mixture of thirty herbs and spices, and has a warm mellow flavour which is particularly pleasant when the drink is served warm. It is based on a medieval Benedictine recipe and is produced at Welle Manor Hall at Upwell in Norfolk.

Country Wines

The main ingredients for traditional country wines have often been flowers, leaves or berries that also have many other uses. Once you have located some good hedges in your area, or established some traditional plants in your garden, you will have supplies that will meet many requirements. The following plants are all popular for country wine-making.

Blackberries are good for red wine and also provide dietary fibre when used as a dessert or in jams. The leaves can be used for tea, and an infusion of leaves and berries can be taken as an antidote for diarrhoea. The berries are a good source of vitamin A, and also some vitamin C.

Dandelion heads can be used for wine, the leaves can be added to salads, and the roots can be roasted for coffee. If your garden is mainly for produce, they are an asset rather than a problem.

Roses are particularly versatile. The petals are used for wine, crystallisation and fragrance. The hips are a rich source of vitamin C, and they can be used for jellies, puddings and even soups.

Sloes are good for wine, sloe gin, and as a supply of 'ink' for linens. The berries are a beautiful colour, and the delicate blossom blends well into a mixed hedge.

Elder trees supply produce for a large part of the year but if you use the same hedge frequently from which to pluck your flowers, you will reduce your supply of berries — so plan how to pick your 'crop'. The flowers can be used for 'champagne', for fritters, and in various summer drinks. The berries can be used for wine, jams and jellies, and as a dessert (alone or with apples). Medicinally, elder is used mainly for colds and sore throats.

The 'haws' from hawthorn can be used to make jelly suitable for use with savoury dishes (a little like rowan jelly). They also make a light rose wine, and are valued by herbalists as a remedy for heart and circulation problems.

Nettles can be cooked to provide a vegetable similar to spinach, also to flavour soup. They are frequently used in wine, occasionally for nettle beer. They can be used in hair rinses, and are valued medicinally as a remedy for anaemia.

The following recipes are for a selection of wines: light white (dandelion), rosé (hawthorn), dry red (sloe) and full red (elderberry).

Dandelion

Items required

6 pints dandelion heads	1 oz bruised root ginger
1 gallon water	8 ozs raisins
4 lbs sugar	1 sachet of all-purpose wine
2 lemons	yeast

Preparation

1. Put the flowers into a container (this could be a white plastic bucket covered by a cloth) and pour in the boiling water.
2. Leave for three days, stirring occasionally.
3. Strain into a pan, add sugar, lemon rind and ginger. Bring to the boil and simmer for half an hour.
4. Cool and strain into a demijohn. Add the raisins, lemon juice and yeast.
5. Ferment, rack (syphon into a fresh demijohn, leaving any sediment behind), and keep for one year when bottled.

Hawthorn

Items required

6 lbs haws	3 lbs sugar
1 gallon water	1 sachet of all-purpose wine
	yeast

Preparation

1. Put the haws into a container and pour in the boiling water.

2. Leave covered and untouched for 5-6 weeks.
3. Remove the scum from the surface and strain off the liquid.
4. Add the sugar, bring to the boil, and simmer for half an hour.
5. Cool, add the yeast, and pour into a demijohn.
6. Top up to one gallon with cool boiled water, and leave to ferment.
7. Rack and leave for several months before drinking.

Sloe

Items required

4 lbs ripe sloes	1 lemon
1 gallon water	2 lbs sugar
8 ozs raisins	1 sachet Burgundy wine yeast

Preparation

1. Prick or cut the sloes and put into a container. Pour in the boiling water and leave for several days.
2. Strain off the liquid, add the raisins, sliced lemon and sugar. Bring to the boil and simmer for half an hour.
3. Cool, add yeast, and pour into a demijohn.
4. Ferment, rack and bottle. Keep for at least six months.

Elderberry

Items required

2 pints elderberries (stalks removed — this can be done by pulling a fork through the berries)	3 lbs sugar
	1 cup strong cold tea
	1 oz bruised root ginger
	1 sachet of Burgundy wine yeast
1 gallon water	

Preparation

1. Put the berries into a pan. Add the water and bring to the boil.
2. Simmer for about half an hour, then strain and add the sugar.
3. Cool, then add the tea, ginger and yeast. Pour into a demijohn.
4. Top up to one gallon with cool boiled water. Leave to ferment for 3-4 weeks.

5. Rack into a clean demijohn and ferment for another 3 months.
6. Bottle and keep for about 1 year.

Sloe Gin

Items required

12 ozs sloes   1 bottle of gin
4 ozs sugar

Preparation

1. Prick or cut the sloes and put them into a jar large enough to hold the gin, sloes and sugar. Use a dark jar or store the jar in a dark place.
2. Mix the gin and sugar, then pour the mixture over the sloes.
3. Seal the jar and shake it gently.
4. Leave for three months, shaking occasionally.
5. Strain off the liquid and keep for a further three months.

Pecheur

This is a French drink, otherwise known as 'La Biere Amoreuse'. It is produced by Fischer of Strasbourg. Ingredients include ginseng, ginger, cardamon and myrtle. Unlike other beers, it is regarded as an aphrodisiac.

If you have tried Pecheur and enjoyed it, or would like to make your own herb-flavoured beer, make a list of the herbs you might enjoy with hops and add them to a brew of your own.

Angostura Bitters

'Bitters' have been used in England since the end of the eighteenth century. Originally, they were flavoured with Angostura (*Galipea cuspara*), named after the town of Angostura (now Ciudad Bolivar) in Venezuela. Today they are flavoured with yellow gentian (*Gentiana lutea*) but the name remains the same.

Angostura bitters are used in many well-known drinks, particularly cocktails and mixed drinks. The following examples are amongst the most popular:

Pink Gin

3 dashes Angostura bitters
1 measure gin

1 measure water
ice

Manhattan

1 measure whisky
½ measure vermouth
1 dash Angostura bitters

ice
lemon

Rob Roy

1 measure whisky
1 measure vermouth
1 dash Angostura bitters

ice
maraschino cherry

Whisky 'Old Fashioned'

1 dash Angostura bitters
1 cube sugar
ice

1 measure of whisky
1 maraschino cherry
dash or two of soda.

Angostura bitters are also used in soups and stews to give a pungent, slightly sharp taste. They are part of a group of liquid herb mixes which include Tabasco, the flavouring used sparingly in dishes such as Chili Con Carne. Tabasco is made from spirit vinegar, red pepper and salt.

Changing food fashions have given rise to various new liquid herb mixes suitable for use in such things as stir fried dishes and barbecues where quickly absorbed flavourings are an advantage. One range of liquid herbs is produced by Rayners.

Herb Flavoured Oils and Vinegars

These provide a blend of herb flavours and liquid for a range of culinary purposes. Herb flavoured vinegars are particularly suitable for savoury dishes, dressings, and preserves. Herb flavoured oils can be used for frying, grilling, salad dressings, gravies and sauces. Both types of liquid look very attractive when carefully prepared and kept.

Flavoured vinegars need to be steeped for 2-3 weeks before use. They should be kept in plastic bottles with plastic lids. Avoid using metal lids or metal spoons for mixing. If no suitable bottles are available, use glass jars and cover with cling-film. They can steep in a sunny place but should be stored in a cool, dark place when ready.

Use white wine vinegar and fresh undamaged herbs. Pick the herbs before flowering when they are at their most aromatic. The best herb vinegars are usually mint, lavender, French tarragon, borage, thyme and red basil. An additional flavour popular for sauces is raspberry. This requires a slightly different method.

Raspberry vinegar

Items required

6 ozs raspberries
12 fl ozs white wine vinegar

Preparation

1. Crush the raspberries, add to the vinegar, and leave for four days.
2. Strain and bottle.
3. Keep for about one month before use.

All of these herb vinegars last for about a year. If kept longer, try a small amount to check that they have not deteriorated.

Flavoured oils can be made in a similar way. Olive or sunflower oil produce the best results. When the herbs have been added, leave them to steep for a couple of weeks on a sunny shelf or sill. When they are ready, store them in a cool, dark cupboard.

Food Colourings from Herbs

Two of the best-known herb colourings are saffron and turmeric.

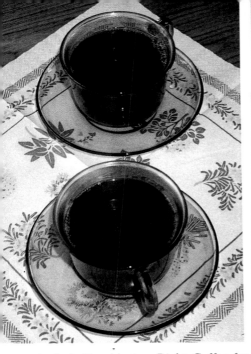
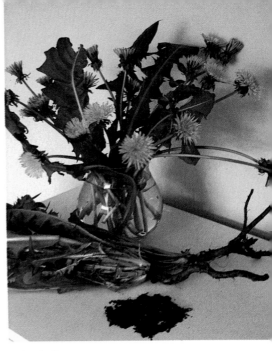

△ *Left*: Rosehip tea. *Right*: Coffee from dandelion roots.

▽ *Left*: Hawthorn wine during the early stages. *Right*: Angostura bitters and liquid herbs.

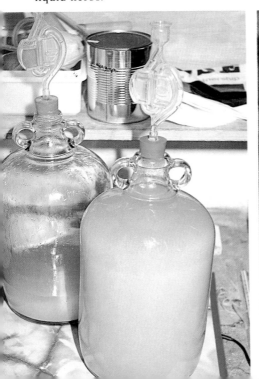
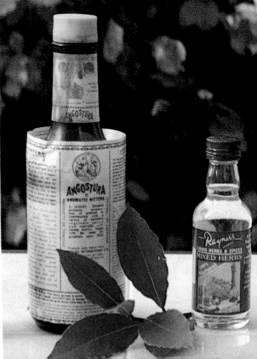

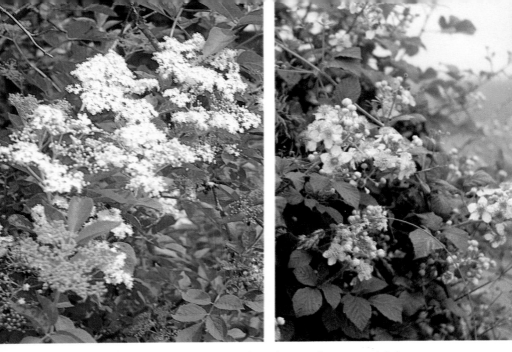

△ *Left*: Elder flowers and berries for wines and summer drinks.
Right: Blackberry — leaves for teas, berries for wines and dyes.

▽ *Left*: Sunflower — for sunflower oil. *Right*: Heather for fabric dyes.

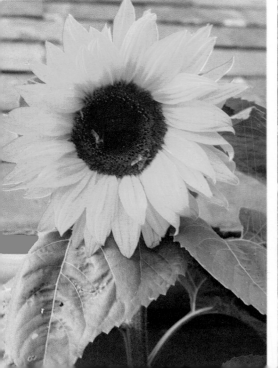

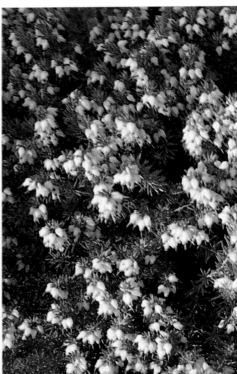

Saffron (*Crocus sativus*) is most often used to colour rice for use with light meat dishes, and for paella. It also gives the distinctive colour to Cornish saffron cakes.

Turmeric (*Curcuma longa*) is used to give curries their orange/yellow shades. Unlike saffron, it is also used as a fabric dye.

Fabric Colourings from Herbs

Our modern chemical dyes started to replace traditional dyes during the last century. Until then, dyes were produced from a range of natural substances which tended to produce more subtle colours than their early chemical rivals. Occasional comments in Victorian novels or newspapers describe the rather harsh new colours to be seen alongside traditional ones such as dark reds, greens or browns.

If you try some traditional dyeing herbs, it will mostly be the more subtle colours that you create — colours from natural substances that retain an earthy, sunlit glow. You will need quite large amounts of plants, and if you want the colours to be permanent, you will also need to use a mordant. This will usually be alum, tin, iron, or chrome. Alum is the most frequently used of these substances.

Wool is the easiest material to dye in this way but the mixture needs to be boiled and this will shrink the wool. For this reason, the thread should be dyed and not completed articles.

The plants can be used fresh or dried. Many hedgerow plants can be picked as required but permission may be necessary before digging roots unless you can grow your own plants. Dried plants and mordants can be obtained from craft shops. The following plants can all be used with an alum mordant:

Plant	*Colour*
Onion skins (*Allium cepa*)	light brown
Bracken roots (*Pteris aquilina*)	orange
Tansy flowers (*Tanacetum vulgare*)	yellow
Birch leaves (*Betula pendula*)	yellow
Heather shoots (*Calluna vulgaris*)	yellow/beige
Elder leaves (*Sambucus nigra*)	green
Elder berries (*Sambucus nigra*)	mauve
Blackberries (*Rubus fructicosus*)	grey

To dye wool with one of these plants, use the following method:

First process

Items required

8 ozs alum   2 lbs wool thread
2 ozs cream of tartar   water
(obtainable from craft shops —
different from baking tartar)

Preparation

1. Put the water, alum and tartar into the dyeing containers. Allow sufficient water to cover the wool easily.
2. Mix and bring to the boil.
3. Add the wool and simmer for half an hour.
4. Remove the wool and squeeze out the excess water.

Second process

Items required

Prepared wool   water
2 lbs plant material   muslin bag

Preparation

1. Put the plant material and the wool into the muslin bag and add sufficient water to cover easily.
2. Bring the ingredients to the boil.
3. Simmer for one hour.
4. Remove the wool and rinse it in clear water.

Inks

The juice from sloes (*Prunus spinosa*) provides an ink for use on linens. And the juice from Poke root berries (*Phytolacca americana*) provides an ink for use on paper.

A Scent of Herbs

Fragrance is an elusive but potent quality. Some perfumes can be recognised after many years even though the scent they create varies from person to person. They are like melodies with variations, recognisable yet individual.

Flowers are a major source of fragrance, and over the years many techniques have evolved for extracting and fixing their scents. The rarity of great perfumes in the past — due mainly to the difficulties of producing them — ensured that successful ones became very well-known. Some are still famous today. Hungary Water with its base of rosemary dates from the fourteenth century, Eau-de-Cologne from the eighteenth century. The latter also includes rosemary but alongside other herbs such as lemon balm, coriander and orange blossom.

Two of the most frequently used flower fragrances are rose and lavender. Attar of roses is one of the oldest known perfumes. Lavender was popular by Roman times and continues to be in use today.

Certain areas, where conditions were particularly suitable for the growing of fragrant plants, have given their names to particular products. Others have become centres for the manufacture of perfume.

Lavender fields have been established in Provence for centuries. Items from the early years of the perfume trade of that area can be seen in Grasse at the Musée d'Art et d'Histoire de Provence. Local scent factories such as Molinard and Fragonard are also open to visitors.

English lavender has long been used for perfumes and references to English lavender water date back to the twelfth century. Today the largest area of commercially grown lavender is at Heacham in Norfolk. In the past, lavender fields were mainly concentrated in and around London. Lavender sold abroad was sometimes known as

Mitcham lavender; now only streets with names such as Lavender Avenue give a clue to Mitcham's past. Similarly, lavender has long ceased to be grown near Lavender Hill in London. But even if the plants have been moved elsewhere, many products remain the same. Yardley's lavender water has been on sale since the eighteenth century.

The names of some roses also give clues to their use and popularity in certain areas. *Rosa gallica officinalis* is sometimes known as Apothecary's rose or Provins rose, reflecting its medicinal uses and the rose fields where it grew, at Provins near Paris.

Although the rose has been grown in many countries, it has particularly strong associations with England. As the national flower, appearing on coins, sport strips, buildings and logos, it is seen throughout the country. For this reason, and others, it is quite surprising that the rose oil market is currently dominated by other European countries. In Yorkshire, Dr. Peter Wilde is trying to remedy this. His rose farm is already producing oil, and the first product — luxury soap — is on the market.

Dr. Wilde is concentrating on what he calls 'boudoir products' but rose, and other essential oils, have a wide range of therapeutic uses as well. They can be used either for self-help at home, or with the guidance of a professional trained in one of the relevant therapies.

Aromatherapy

The link between particular fragrances and feelings or health have long been recognised. The ancient Egyptians used various fragrant substances for healing, and it was partly the scent that gave lotus flowers such significance in Egyptian culture.

Over the years, these links have been investigated more systematically. Earlier this century, a French chemist, Professor Gattefosse, first used the term *aromatherapy* to describe the use of essential oils for healing.

Essential oils carry the fragrance of plants. They are normally obtained by a process of distillation. For storage and sale, the oil is then diluted in a carrier such as alcohol or vegetable oil. The mixture is then sold in small bottles with droppers. Some oils can be very expensive but only tiny amounts are used at a time. Prices vary from £2 or £3 for 10 ml of lavender or lemon to about £12 for frankincense, and as much as £50 for orange blossom or rose absolute.

Aromatherapists are available if you would like professional advice about this form of therapy. Information can be obtained from:

The International Federation of Aromatherapists,
46 Dalkieth Road,
London SE21.

It is also possible to treat various common ailments at home. For this purpose, oils for inhalation, bathing and massage are usually recommended. Oils should only be taken internally on the advice of a qualified aromatherapist. If you find it difficult to obtain oils, try one of the suppliers listed in Chapter 9.

At home, oils can be used in the following ways, unless otherwise stated on the container:

Inhalation

Boil about one pint of water, then leave to cool for a few minutes. Add about 3-5 drops of oil, then inhale the evaporating oil.

Bathing

Add five or six drops to the water when you are ready.

Massage

Add four or five drops of oil to ½ cup of carrier oil (e.g. soya oil).

Each oil has a particular purpose. You can check this with your suppliers, for example: basil for nervousness, orange blossom for depression or stress, lavender to calm and rosemary to stimulate. Certain oils are also recommended for various common ailments: pine oil for bronchitis, lemon oil as a sedative, thyme oil for fatigue and fennel oil for digestion. In some cases, blends of several oils may be used for a particular purpose.

The Bach Flower Remedies

These provide a similar system which is ideal for practice at home. Their aim is to heal by enhancing harmony between mind and body. They were developed by Dr. Edward Bach (1886-1936) who worked in orthodox medicine but gradually developed his own plant therapy. For example, mustard, larch, pine and elm are part of the group for relieving various aspects of depression or anguish. Water violet, heather and impatiens are for loneliness. There are also various combined remedies. These include 'Rescue Remedy' and 'Grief Mix'.

For further details of the remedies, contact:

Dr. Edward Bach Centre,
Mount Vernon,
Sotwell,
Wallingford,
Oxon.

Some Traditional Herb Products

Traditional fragrant items such as pot pourri and pomanders developed at a time when they were regarded as fumigants as well as scents. Insect-repellant herbs were strewn over floors with rushes, sachets were kept amongst clothes, and furniture smelled of herbs and beeswax. For a hint of nostalgia, try some of the following.

Pot Pourri

Pot pourri is an attractive addition to any household. It can have a dominant fragrance or colour to suit the mood of each room, or a single mixture can be used throughout the house.

You might enjoy a bowl of pot pourri beside your favourite chair, or you might have a suitable group of containers for use at points around the house. An example of this approach for many rooms can be seen at Stratfield Saye, home of the Dukes of Wellington. The main rooms each have a pot pourri in an elegant marble container. These provide a gentle breath of summer amongst the history and formality.

In your home, pot pourri could complement particular features or provide a contrast. A rose pot pourri might be suitable for a bedroom with rose-patterned fabrics or paper. A pine pot pourri could be placed beside a window with a distant view of pine woods. An urban flat with no garden could have a window box and nearby pot pourri. Each room or feature will suggest a possible design or flower.

If you have little time it is possible to buy pot pourri. Some attractive mixtures are available, but the fragrance is rarely as good as that from a home-made one. Most bought mixtures rely on the addition of particular oils. These usually give a stronger but less subtle fragrance than a blend from your own selection of flowers.

If you have time to make your own pot pourri, there are two main types of mixtures: dry and moist. The first will produce the most attractive mixture, the second is the traditional method and will give a longer-lasting fragrance. The name, pot pourri, comes from this second method. It means 'rotten pot' and refers to the rotting petals and leaves of the moist method.

When you have decided which method to use, consider whether you would like a dominant fragrance or a blend. Traditionally, most pot pourris have had a base of rose petals or lavender. These keep their scent better than other flowers even if fixatives are not used. However, you may prefer a different base, and fixatives need not be a problem.

In the past, many fragrant products have been fixed, or mixed, with animal substances such as ambergris (from sperm whales), civet (from *Civettictis civetta*), or musk (from the male musk deer). Today, many people avoid these substances in the hope of causing less suffering to the animals concerned. Suitable plant fixatives are such things as orris root (*Iris germanica*), tonquin bean (*Dipteryx odorata*) or gum benzoin (*Styrax officinalis*).

Dry Pot Pourri

Unless you have a large garden with all the flowers you need, you can make the pot pourri from a mixture of bought and collected flowers. Details of suppliers are given in Chapter 9.

Collect fresh flowers and leaves only on a dry day. It is very difficult to dry them successfully if they start off damp. Petals from large flowers should be dried separately. Small flowers can be dried whole. If you pick flowers throughout the summer, some will be ready much earlier than others. These can be stored in paper bags which leave plenty of room for the petals (or leaves) to be gently shaken about now and then. When all the petals and leaves are ready, mix them thoroughly and add the spices with your chosen fixative. Then put the mixture into airtight containers. For large amounts, sweet jars are useful if kept in a dark place. Leave for about a month but shake occasionally.

The mixture should now be ready for display. It should last about six months to a year — but if you are reluctant to part with it, add some small amounts of essential oil.

Possible ingredients:

From those listed below, or others that you have checked out, make a selection that will achieve the desired effect. One possible addition, for example, would be pine needles, tiny pine cones and star anise to give a woody effect.

Flowers:

Rose petals and buds, lavender, peony, phlox, clove carnation, honeysuckle, jasmine, hyssop, syringa, rosemary, violet, wallflower, delphinium, marigold.

Leaves:

Basil, bay, myrtle, sage, rosemary, eucalyptus, mint, lemon thyme, lemon balm.

Spices:

Allspice, nutmeg, cinnamon, cloves, coriander, ginger, mace, caraway (grate or crush these).

Fixatives

Various fixatives such as orris root can be obtained from craft shops or the suppliers listed in Chapter 9.

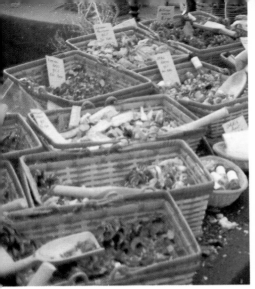 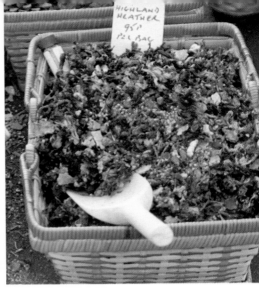

△ *Left*: Pot pourri for sale at a country fair. *Right*: Highland heather pot pourri.

▽ Commercially-available pot pourri (apple).

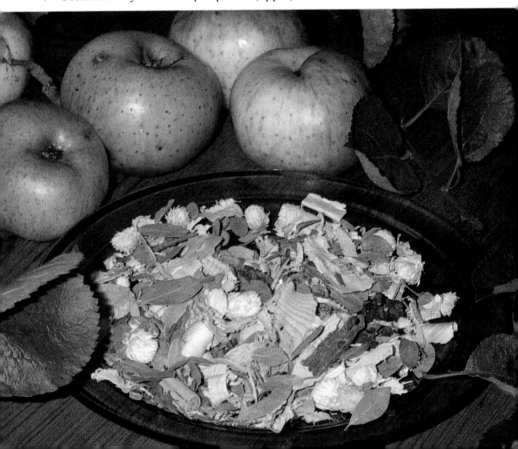

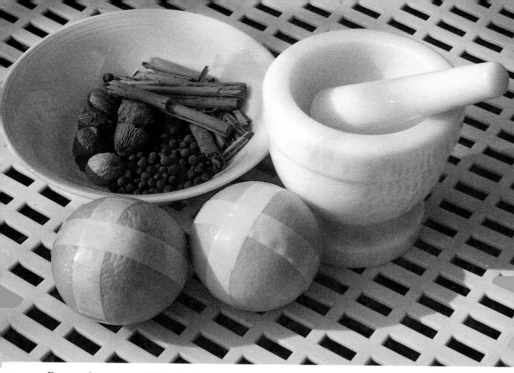

Pomanders: a traditional gift from lovers — see pages 64 and 65 for instructions on how to make them.

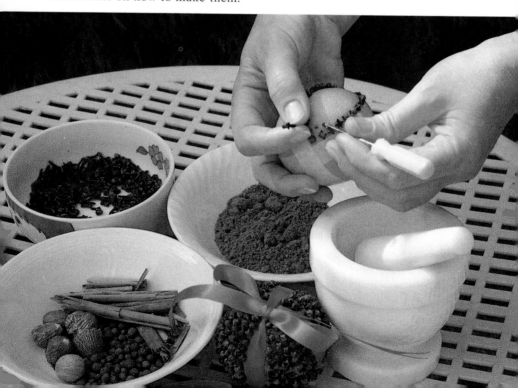

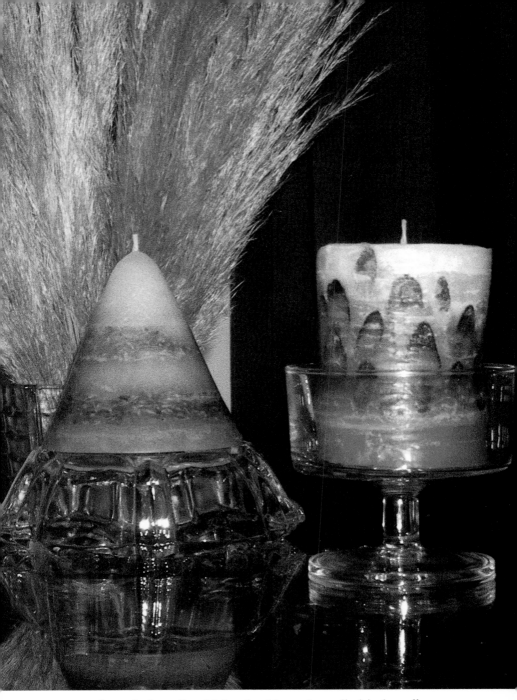

Home-made conical candle with bands of lavender, cylindrical candle
showing decoration of sage leaves.

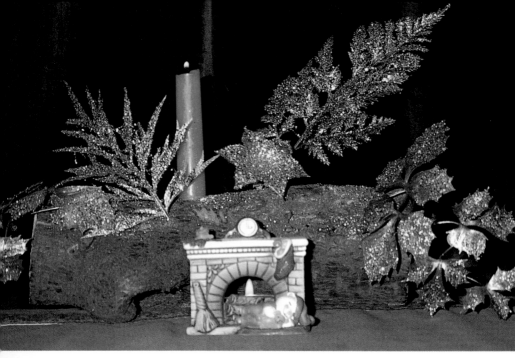

△ Fireplace with commercially-produced bayberry candle.

▽ Herb-scented water candles — fill holders with coloured water, add vegetable oil mixed with essential oil (see chapter five) for fragrance, and place plastic floats and wicks on the oil.

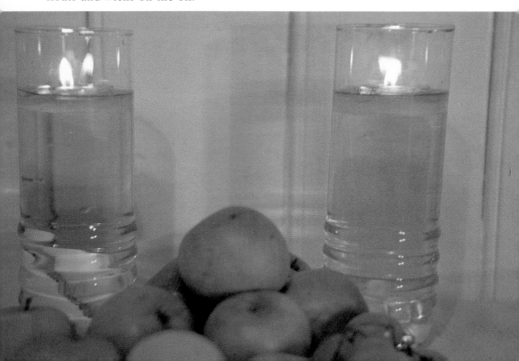

Moist pot pourri

Select your plants and leaves from those listed above or from your own list. As this method involves rotting down the leaves and petals, very woody plants are usually less suitable. However, if you want a particular effect or fragrance, it is always worth experimenting.

When you have decided on the mixture you require, dry each batch as you collect them. Just wait a couple of days, then put the limp plants into a deep bowl or sweet jar (if kept in the dark). Sprinkle each layer with rock salt and press down before adding another layer. When the bowl or jar is full, mix the contents, then leave for a couple of weeks.

Mix again, then add your chosen spices and fixative. Return the mixture to the bowl or jar for several months before use.

Pomanders

These days we use pomanders as decorative air fresheners but they were originally carried around as a protection against airborne infections. Those for the rich were made of costly blends of such things as ambergris, herbs and spices. Some were simply held in the hand, others were kept in ornate containers. Some pomander designs were minor works of art. Various examples in gold and silver can be seen in the Victoria and Albert Museum. They were like an extension of personal perfumes and jewellery, and they featured in quite a few love poems of the sixteenth and seventeenth centuries.

This century has given them fewer romantic associations but they have not completely disappeared from poems. In *The Clove Orange* Eleanor Farjeon celebrates another style of pomander, a citrus fruit studded with cloves — the version of the pomander which is now most often seen. •

'The Clove Orange'

I'll make a clove orange to give to my darling,
I'll make a clove orange to please my delight,
And lay her in her coffer to sweeten her linen,
And hang by her pillow to sweeten her night.

I'll choose a small orange as round as the moon is,
That ripened its cheek in the sunniest grove,
And when it is dry as a Midsummer hayfield
I'll stick it all round with the head of the clove.

To spice the dull sermon in church of a Sunday
Her orange of cloves in her bag she shall take;
When parson is prosy and eyelids are drowsy,
One sniff at her spice-ball will charm her awake.

And when she walks forth in the highways and bye-ways,
Where fevers are prone and infection is rife,
On her palm she shall carry her little Clove Orange,
A charm against sickness, to guard her sweet life.

And moth shall not haunt her most delicate garment,
Nor spectre her delicate dream in the night,
When she hangs in her chamber the little dried orange
I've studded with cloves to delight my Delight.

by Eleanor Farjeon

Pomanders can be made quite easily, particularly using an orange. A lemon is slightly harder to manage. If you would like a bowl of pomanders, rather than one or two to hang up, try limes — or a mixture of oranges and limes.

Pomanders usually have some areas free of cloves. These provide a pattern, and a space for a ribbon — but they are not essential. The method described below is for an orange with ribbons but you might like to try other patterns of your own.

1. Put two bands of sticky tape lightly round the orange so that they cross at the top and bottom.
2. Test the skin. If it is thin and tender, you may be able to press cloves in straightaway. If not, prick holes in the skin before inserting them.
3. Fill the sections between the tapes with cloves. They can make a pattern or be placed at random.

4. Remove the tape.
5. Mix cinnamon, nutmeg or mixed spices with a fixative such as orris root powder — then shake the mixture all over the oranges.
6. Leave the orange for about a month — it will dry out and shrink a little. Then tie on the ribbons and use.

Herb-scented Candles

Although candles are no longer required for lighting, many households still use them. They may be valued for their colour, scent, or symbolic purpose. Lightly-scented candles might be required for a dinner-party — Christmas candles might burn down to reveal pine needles and an aroma of frankincense.

If you are making herb-scented candles, consider their purpose and the likely holder before finalising your design. For simple candle-making you require: a mould, paraffin wax, stearine, wicks and herbs. It is easiest to make candles using simple materials from a craft shop and adding herb scents or decorations as required.

The mould

If you intend to make candles regularly, a selection of moulds is useful. If not — tins, cartons, even bottles (if not required again) will serve the same purpose. With bottles, you will need to wrap the bottled candle in newspaper, smash the glass, and withdraw the candle.

If you are using a mould, oil it before starting. Also, unless it is to be broken or peeled off, ensure that the open end is wider than the closed end.

It is possible to make candles without moulds by using the dipping method. But this takes longer and makes it more difficult to add decorative herbs.

The wick

Tie one end of the wick round a pencil or twig and balance it across the open end of the mould. If you can make a tiny hole in the bottom of the mould, pull the other end of the wick through it. If not, weight the loose end with a washer or something similar.

The wax

Paraffin wax is the simplest material to use. It melts at around 55° C (you can use a confectionary thermometer if you wish). Some additives such as stearine can also be used if a more resilient or shiny candle is required. You can also melt down old candles.

For coloured candles, oil-soluble dyes are available but some good results can be obtained simply using the natural colour decorated with herbs.

Melt the wax in a saucepan with a pouring lip — for small moulds a metal funnel might also be useful.

The herbs

You can produce a decorated and fragrant candle by adding whole sprigs to wax as it is poured into the mould. Lavender and rosemary are good for this. Chopped or powdered herbs can also be added, or a few drops of essential oil.

Some herbs have long associations with candlemaking but these are not necessarily the best ones to use at home. Bayberry (*Myrica cerifera*) is also known as waxberry or candleberry. A scented fat is obtained from the plant for candlemaking. It is a popular fragrance for commercially produced scented candles but it requires a good supply of plants and time for an additional process before home-candlemaking can begin.

Some interesting and original results can be obtained from experiments with herbs from your own garden. Additional herbs, spices, and essential oils can be added to suit personal tastes. You could, for example, place sprigs of your own herb round the mould for decoration and mild fragrance, then add essential oil of the same or a complementary fragrance.

Scented Plants for the Garden and House

If space permits, you may want to set aside an area of your garden for scented plants. If you have little space, window boxes can provide miniature gardens, or containers can bring some outdoor scents indoors.

A fragrant garden is a good source of plants for such things as pot pourri as well as a source of more immediate pleasure. Planning will involve the best use of the space available, and the best combination of fragrances with some note of the seasons when flowers or leaves are at their most aromatic.

Many people have a favourite flower fragrance which evokes pleasant memories, creates a calm mood, or is particularly refreshing. If, for example, you like honeysuckle, you could set out an area of cream or white scented plants, perhaps including one or two for other purposes: broom or white buddleia would attract bees and butterflies.

If the rose is your favourite flower, you could select those with a special colour or fragrance, or you might concentrate on old-fashioned varieties. Many roses have interesting histories and associations.

It is possible to buy various species of wild roses such as *Rosa xanthina* which originated in the Far East, or *Rosa dupontii* (named after Andre Dupont, a nineteenth century director of the Luxembourg Gardens in Paris).

The group of roses known as the gallicas almost certainly includes the first roses cultivated by man. If you are interested in this group, examples include: *Rosa gallica versicolour*, also known as *Rosa Mundi*. It is said to have been named after Fair Rosamond, mistress of Henry II.

Damask roses include *Rosa damascena versicolour*, the York and Lancaster rose. This group of roses is also very old — they are strongly scented and suitable for pot pourri. They are also frequently used for attar of roses.

Another long-established group is the Albas. They are not white as the name suggests but usually pink. They include *Rosa alba maxima*, otherwise known as Bonnie Prince Charlie's rose.

These, and other traditional roses, have become more popular in recent years. Some can be obtained from local garden centres, others are available from specialist suppliers as listed in Chapter 9.

There are certain herbs with unexpected fragrances and these can make an interesting small group. Pineapple sage really does smell of pineapple. Lemon thyme and lemon balm smell strongly of lemon. Fennel leaves smell of aniseed, and rue has a very individual peppery fragrance which has been described as resembling a host of different things.

If you are looking for some new plants try to check as many features as possible before you buy them. If you are browsing through herb catalogues, take a quick look at the latin names. Herbs valued for their fragrance often have *fragrans* or *odorata* for their second name.

A Touch of Herbs

Herbal products to heal, cleanse and perfume have a long history. Many were made at home for family use. A well-stocked household might include such things as soapwort shampoo, beeswax polish, comfrey ointment and rosewater. Some herbs have names indicating their usefulness for such purposes: soapwort (*Saponaria officinalis*), eyebright (*Euphrasia officinalis*), and bottlebrush (*Equisetum arvense*), for example.

Products for sale — often with secret recipes — were once made only in certain places. Hungary Water, Eau de Cologne and English lavender water derived their names from their original places of manufacture. Their popularity encouraged the establishment of businesses for the commercial production of popular fragrances. One or two of these companies remain in business today.

Yardley's first product in 1770 was soap — perfumed with lavender. Another popular product at the time was 'Bear's Grease', useful for keeping hair and wigs tidy! The list of items gradually increased — by the 1880s a New York stockist offered twenty-two varieties of Yardley's soap for sale. These included 'Elder Flower' and 'Otto Rose' as well as the famous 'Old Brown Windsor'. The range of products continued to grow but lavender was never eclipsed. As the company moved into the twentieth century, it became the largest manufacturer of lavender products in the world. Supplies of lavender from fields around London declined as the city grew but demand for Yardley's 'Old English Lavender' products continued to increase. These days the lavender is grown in Norfolk.

With time, new plants and products have joined the traditional repertoire. Aloe (*Aloe vera*) and jojoba (*Simmondsia chinensis*) are now popular ingredients in natural cosmetics. Exotic and once rare perfumes such as patchouli and neroli can be obtained without difficulty. A fragrance or effect is now available to suit most tastes.

Due partly to worries about chemicals and animal testing, natural cosmetics have also become increasingly popular. Various suppliers, including the Body Shop offer simple products such as plain 'vegetable soap'. Potter's supply a range of 'Skin Clear' products, and large stores now stock various groups of natural cosmetics.

It is also possible to make quite a wide range of natural cosmetics and household cleansers for yourself. Consider some of the fragrances you most enjoy for personal and home use; many recipes can be adapted to include your favourite fragrance.

Bodycare

When making any of the following items, use stainless steel or enamel vessels if boiling is required.

Simple preparations from herbs and water

Hair rinses

Make an infusion (see page 88) using a suitable herb. Strain the liquid and add it to the water for the final rinsing of the hair. Rosemary can be used for any hair type. To heighten fair hair, try camomile. For dark hair, try sage. Greasy hair will benefit from lavender, dry hair from comfrey.

Fragrant steaming

Useful for softening and toning the skin of the face and neck. Choose one or more herbs with a fragrance you enjoy. Put about a handful of the dried herbs into a large basin or bowl. Pour one or two pints of boiling water over the herbs — then lean over the bowl for five to ten minutes while covering your head and shoulders with a towel. Arrange the towel so that it traps as much steam as possible.

Rose Water

Other fragrant petals such as elder, violet, rosemary or honeysuckle can also be used in this way.

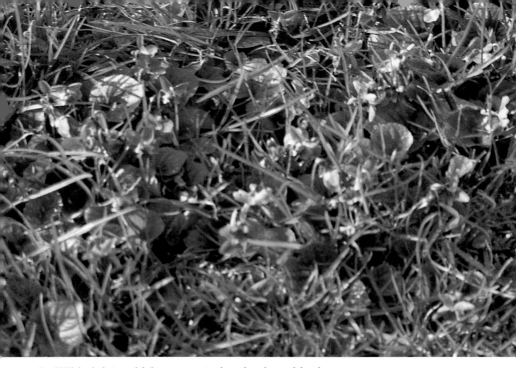

△ Wild violets add fragrance to hand gels and baths.

▽ Marigold petals for a face lotion.

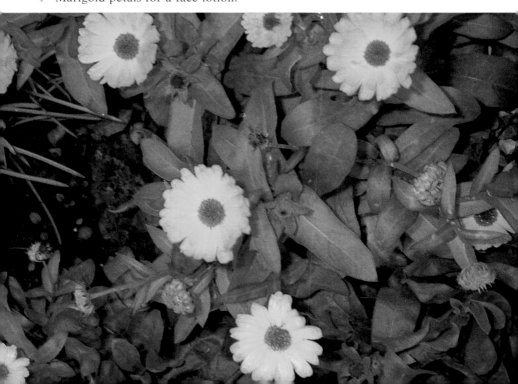

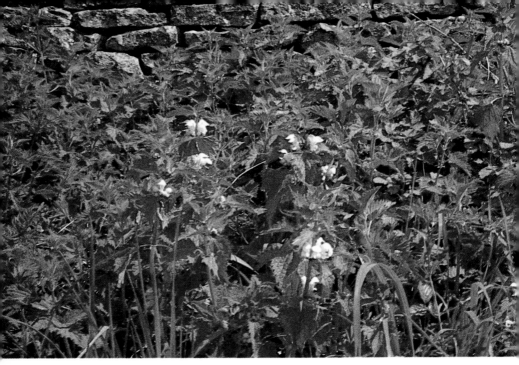

△ Nettle tea is beneficial to the skin.

▽ Essential oils.

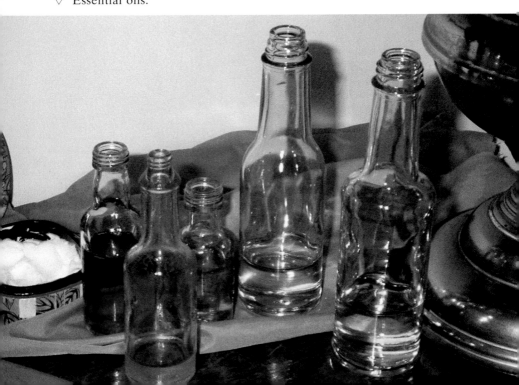

Ingredients

1 pint rose petals
1 pint distilled water
1 teaspoon borax

Preparation

1. Rinse the rose petals, then pulp them in a blender.
2. Put the pulp into a saucepan, add the distilled water, and bring to the boil.
3. Simmer for two or three minutes, and add the borax.
4. Pour the mixture into a clear bottle and leave to stand on a window-sill for a few days.
5. Strain, bottle, and keep in a cool place.

Lotions

Marigold Face Lotion

Ingredients

8 fl ozs distilled water
handful of marigold petals
1½ teaspoons almond oil

a pinch of borax
1 teaspoon glycerine

Preparation

1. Put the marigold petals into a bowl deep enough for whisking.
2. Boil the water and pour it over the petals.
3. Add the glycerine and almond oil drop by drop while whisking.
4. Continue whisking while adding the borax.
5. Leave to cool.
6. Strain before bottling. Keep in a cool place.

Rose Body Lotion

This lotion can also be made with other suitable flower waters (see page 70).

Ingredients

½ pint rosewater
2 tablespoons glycerine
a few drops of essential oil

Preparation

1. Heat the rosewater to boiling.
2. Add the glycerine drop by drop while whisking.
3. Continue whisking while adding the essential oil.
4. Leave to cool.
5. Bottle.

Lemon Hand Cream

Ingredients

6 tablespoons lanolin
4 tablespoons vegetable oil
a few drops of lemon oil

Preparation

1. Heat the lanolin gently in a bowl over hot water — just until it melts.
2. Heat the vegetable oil to the same temperature.
3. Whisk the oil into the lanolin.
4. As it starts to thicken, remove from the heat but continue whisking.
5. Add the lemon oil.
6. Leave to cool.

Gels

Violet Hand Gel

The fragrance of violets — wild or cultivated — has been admired for centuries. Like other popular plants, they became associated with particular areas, sometimes misleadingly. Cultivated Parma violets are well-known but violet-scented products from Parma in Italy were often not made from violets at all but from orris root (*Iris florentina*) which has a similar fragrance.

In the nineteenth century, when violet cultivation became established around Grasse, in Provence, orris root was still used. Soon after that time, when it became easier to extract the perfume from violet flowers due to technical advances, it also happened that two German scientists identified the chemical composition of the fragrance from orris root. In these ways, and others, the history and uses of the two plants have often come together.

In this country, violet fields were established around London and in the West Country. The fields around London disappeared due to urbanisation but those in the West Country have remained. Although often referred to as 'Devon Violets', anyone living in the West Country knows that they grow throughout the area.

Those who have followed Derek Tangye's journey along *The Way To Minack* will know that they can be found around Lamorna. The first time I travelled to a talk by Derek Tangye, I went by train from Exeter to Truro, passing the Holcombe violet fields along the way.

Stratford-on-Avon was another area known for its violets, possibly inspiring lines such as:

When daisies pied and violets blue
And lady-smocks all silver-white
And cuckoo-buds of yellow hue
Do paint the meadows with delight.
Love's Labour's Lost, Shakespeare

Wild violets (*Viola odorata*) are valued for various properties including use as a cough remedy but they are probably best-known for their colour and fragrance. Their mucilage content makes them useful for gels.

Ingredients

2 handfuls of fresh violet
  leaves and flowers
½ pint water (violet water if
  you have it)

2 tablespoons glycerine
pinch of borax
a few drops of lavender oil

Preparation

1. Boil the violets gently in the water for about ½ hour.
2. Strain off the liquid and allow to cool a little.
3. Warm the glycerine and whisk it into the liquid.
4. Add the borax and oil while continuing to whisk.
5. Allow to cool, then pour into jars.

Rosemary Skin Gel

First make some rosemary water using the recipe on pages 70 and 73.

Ingredients

1 oz dried Irish moss (Carragheen)	2 tablespoons glycerine
½ pint rosemary water	2 teaspoons borax
	A few drops of rosemary oil

Preparation

1. Soak the Irish moss in the rosemary water for ½ hour.
2. Bring to the boil and simmer for ½ hour.
3. Cool, then strain.
4. Gently heat the glycerine and stir in the borax.
5. Whisk the glycerine into the gel.
6. Add the rosemary oil while whisking.

Homecare

Insect Repellants

The following plants can be grown indoors, on windowsills or by doorways to help repel insects: basil, tansy, rosemary, southernwood and rue.

Moth Deterrents

Fill small muslin bags with a blend of strong herbs and spices — then place the bags in cupboards and drawers. Mix a blend you enjoy as the fragrance may linger slightly on your belongings. Strongly scented spices such as cinnamon and cloves can be added to a blend which includes herbs such as rosemary or sage. Add some orris root to preserve the fragrance — the moths will hate it!

Woodwork Cleanser

This is suitable for woodwork ignored for some time (but which will then be polished):
4 fl ozs real turpentine
4 fl ozs raw linseed oil
4 fl ozs vinegar
1 fl oz methylated spirit

Polish

Most traditional polishes include beewax. Used alone it does not work well. As part of a mixture, it can produce a fragrant, nourishing polish:
4 ozs beeswax
4 ozs carnauba (from *Copernicia cerifera*)
enough real turpentine to produce a satisfactory mix

If you are making your own household products to avoid using harmful chemicals, you might also be interested in products from 'Ark'. They are available from various stores and supermarkets such as: Tesco, Superdrug, Safeway/Presto, Medicare, Asda, Gateway and Boots.

If you have difficulty obtaining them, contact:
Ark Consumer Products Ltd.,
498-500 Harrow Road,
London W9 3QA.

They currently produce seven environment-friendly household cleaning products: washing powder, liquid detergent, two sizes of washing-up liquid, household cleaner, toilet cleaner and window cleaner. These products are all made without using phosphates, optical brighteners, NTA or EDTA, enzymes or chlorine bleaching agents.

First Aid for Minor Skin Injuries

Cuts and Grazes

Witch hazel (*Hamamelis virginiana*) or a weak solution of lavender oil.

Minor Burns

Apply witch hazel (*Hamamelis virginiana*), an infusion of chickweed (*Stellaria media*), or an infusion of marigold (*Calendula officinalis*).

Sunburn

Dab gently with cottonwool soaked in an infusion of marigold.

Essential Oils for Massage

These oils work in various ways. Their effect is not achieved simply by fragrance. Modern research has shown that substances applied to the skin can have much more than a superficial result. It is thought that part of the effect of massage oils is their action on the nervous system.

Different fragrances have different effects, and you need to choose one suited to the purpose of your massage. For example, some oils stimulate, others sedate.

stimulating oils	*sedating oils*
rosemary	lavender
benzoin	camomile
bergamot	clary sage
black pepper	geranium
camphor	thyme

Personal preference is also important, so choose an oil suited to your purpose which also has a fragrance you enjoy. Check the prices too — they vary greatly from oil to oil.

When you buy your oil, you may find that it is labelled according to its 'note'. This indicates the rate of evaporation. High notes evaporate quickly, low notes last.

In massage the oil is also used to help the hands move easily. Only small amounts are required. The oil will usually be in a vegetable oil carrier — pure oils are very rarely used neat on the skin.

Preparing for a massage

The massage may be for a specific purpose or for general relaxation. If you are using massage with a partner, it helps if you are both feeling fairly calm. Do not rush in from a stressful activity leaving little time to prepare. Take a relaxing bath or sit and chat for a while first. A massage can benefit the person who gives it as well as the recipient.

Choose somewhere warm and comfortable for your massage. To avoid problems with the oil, lie on towels or covers that can easily be washed. Cover any cushions you require.

Pour the oil onto your hands and rub them together before touching your partner. Otherwise the touch of the oil might be cold or uncomfortable.

Consider the purpose of the massage before you start and adapt your movements to suit it. Swift, short strokes would be stimulating. Long leisurely strokes could lead to sleep. After several massages, you could try a wider range of strokes and some heavier, kneading movements.

Starting the massage

Decide whether you will massage the whole body or just certain parts. If you are massaging the whole body, keep in mind some order in which you will move from part to part.

The links from the back to all parts of the body make it a good area to massage, and a good place to start a whole massage. The movements can alleviate backache and help reduce stress and tension.

Many people also experience tension in the neck and shoulders, particularly if their job involves sitting or standing for long periods. A soothing massage can help to reduce this.

To massage the face and head, it is best to stand behind your partner who should be lying down. The skin in this area can feel uncomfortable unless your movements follow its natural direction. This is particularly important around the eyes and mouth, for example. Do not use too much oil around the ears, nose, eyes and mouth.

Make sure that the head is comfortable, and not in a position that would make your movements awkward, before massaging the chest and neck.

Vary the pressure as you massage the arms. Try not to press too heavily on the skin over the bones. This could be uncomfortable for your partner. Give some attention to the wrist before massaging the hands. The style of massage for the hands will vary according to your partner's work and age.

The abdomen requires gentle movements and careful attention. You can then move towards the legs. If your partner has a very active lifestyle, or enjoys strenuous exercise, your treatment of the legs will need to be very different to that for a person with a sedentary lifestyle. As you reach the feet, vary your approach to take account of their condition.

As the massage progresses, vary your style and movements. Stroking, circling and kneading can be used with more variations as your experience increases. Always take note of the reactions of your partner and vary your approach in tune with the response.

Other Essential Oils

In addition to oils with a single fragrance, such as cypress, basil, hyssop or thyme, some health shops and branches of Boots now stock Dr. Jean Valnet's blends of essential oils. Dr. Valnet is well-known in France for his interest in phytotherapy (the study of the healing properties of plants).

His blend called Tegarome (lavender, cypress, rosemary, sage, geranium, thyme, and eucalyptus) is particularly useful for sunburn and minor wounds. Another blend, Climarome, can be inhaled to help clear respiratory problems, and Babibad is a relaxing blend for children's baths.

Internal Aids to External Well-being

Herbal Remedies

Various herbs can be taken internally for their general 'cleansing' action which can be beneficial to the skin. The following could be taken morning and evening:

a decoction of burdock root

an infusion of nettle leaves

an infusion of red clover flowerheads

Brewer's Yeast

This comes from hops and is a by-product of brewing — hence its name. It is a natural source of B vitamins which help maintain healthy skin, teeth and bones. It is available in powder or tablet form. Quite a few people prefer the tablets as the taste of the powder is not too pleasant.

Zinc

Zinc has proved useful in reducing acne. It occurs naturally in shellfish such as oysters, also in milk, eggs, nuts and some vegetables such as onions and broccoli. Tablets can also be obtained to supplement a general diet.

Royal Jelly

A rich source of B vitamins which is possibly why it is recommended as an antidote to various skin conditions such as acne.

Evening Primrose Oil

Also recommended for skin problems, particularly acne.

Traditional Remedies

Wayside Dock: For burns and nettle stings.

Lemon: A good skin softener. Can be used on corns. Cover the corn with lemon, then bind and leave for several hours at a time.

Cucumber: To ease tired eyes.
Witch hazel: For cuts and bruises.
Eyebright: An eyewash for sore eyes.
Raw Potato Slices: For scalds and burns.

Some Books and Addresses

Books

Sensual Massage by Nitya Lacroix (Dorling Kindersley)
The Book of Massage by Lucy Lidell (Ebury Press)
Herbal Cosmetics by Camilla Hepper (Thorsons)
The Body Shop Book by Anita Roddick (Macdonalds) offers
   advice on bodycare.
The Body Shop — Franchising A Philosophy by Gilly McKay and
   Alison Corke (Pan).

Addresses

The Body Shop International PLC,
Hawthorn Road,
Wick,
Littlehampton,
West Sussex BN17 7LR
Will provide details of shops and products.

The Soap Shop,
44 Sidwell Street,
Exeter,
Devon EX4 6NS
Sells natural products which have not been tested on animals. Soap is
the main item with various examples of allied products.

Simply Herbal Skincare,
Murdoch,
Kingsway,
Wilton,
Salisbury SP2 OAW
Supplies herbal products for skincare.

Beauty Without Cruelty Ltd.,
Avebury Avenue,
Tonbridge,
Kent TN9 1TL

Well-known these days — and supplying a wide range of products.

Weleda Ltd.,
Heanor Road,
Ilkeston,
Derbyshire DE7 8DR

Supplies a range of natural toothpastes, often available from health stores.

Images

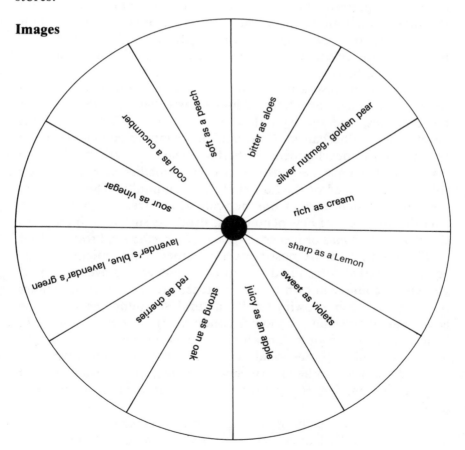

A Cure of Herbs

An increasing number of people now take a serious interest in diet and exercise. Many of them also give careful consideration to the type of treatment they want for particular illnesses. They may use natural remedies as far as possible, or they may rely on orthodox drugs when prescribed by their doctor, and use natural remedies for the many common ailments that can be treated at home. These changes are part of a general movement towards more natural lifestyles in the developed countries, and one result is a new era in the history of herbalism.

If you are interested in herbal remedies, it could be for various reasons. You might be interested in the classic herbals published over the centuries, and the light they throw on past lifestyles and the development of herbalism. Or you might be interested in a particular feature of the development of herbal remedies, perhaps the long tradition of women herbalists dispensing remedies as part of their role as female head of the household or community. Then there are the many unusual stories from the years when there was great rivalry over the discovery of new plant cures. Products such as quinine from *Cinchona officinalis* or ipecac (*Cephaelis ipecacuanha*) brought relief to thousands, and the possibility that other plants might provide equally effective cures lured botanists to danger and even death. If you visit a country known for one of these products, it is sometimes possible to see it growing in its natural surroundings (with the advantage of travelling in today's conditions!). At home, you might be interested in growing plants for your own remedies, or you might want to consult a professional herbalist. Whatever your interest — whether you want to be an armchair herbalist, or you want to start digging and mixing for yourself — a great deal of material is available.

Herbals, guides to the gathering of green remedies, have a long history. The earliest ones were manuscripts based on centuries of knowledge passed on by word of mouth. Probably the most famous and influential of these manuscript herbals was Dioscorides' *De Materia Medica* which dates from the first century A.D. It describes about five hundred plants and gives details of their healing properties. The illustrations are somewhat stylised but it is still possible to identify many of the plants while on holiday in the Mediterranean. There is a copy of the manuscript in Vienna.

In Britain, the best-known manuscript herbal was the *Leech Book of Bald*, which dates from the early tenth century. Bald mentions the work of his fellow *leeches* (doctors) and gives details of remedies that are mainly herbal. Although this is an Anglo-Saxon herbal, it probably reflects work in other areas of Britain, for example, the herbs used by the physicians of Myddfai in Wales.

The information in these manuscript herbals was only gradually superseded during the sixteenth and seventeenth centuries when the first printed herbals became available. From this period come the great herbals of Gerard, Parkinson and Culpeper. Some of their remedies are considered dangerous today, and amongst the reasonable advice there are sprinklings of strange beliefs. However, some of the best known remedies are still used and attract the attention of modern researchers. A recent American study, for example, has shown the action of comfrey on red blood cells. This supports its use for bruises and one of its many descriptive names: *bruisewort.*

The first printed herbals appeared at a time when botany was in its infancy, and herbalism was developing in various directions. Like all herbalists of the time, Gerard reflects these changes in his work. He also included current travellers' tales about plants. These included one about a *tree* believed to grow *geese* in the north of Scotland. But more typical are his comments on the use of roses: 'The conserve of rose. . . taken in the morning fasting, and last at night, strengthneth the heart, and taketh away the shaking and trembling thereof. . .'

The next major herbal to appear was John Parkinson's *Theatrum Botanicum*, published in 1640. Parkinson worked in London and was eventually given the title of Herbalist to Charles I. He owned a shop which he filled with supplies from a nearby garden in Long Acre. His book supplanted Gerard's to some extent and generally gained greater respect. This happened despite doubtful items such as uses for unicorn horn which are given the same attention as traditional (and available!) remedies such as birthwort: 'to help women that are ready to be delivered, and that are delivered. . .'

The third herbalist of this famous trio, Thomas Culpeper, produced a less scholarly but more popular book than his two predecessors. Even today, modern reprints and extracts from his books are more likely to be found in local bookshops. Culpeper worked in Red Lion Street, Spitalfields, London. He was particularly willing to help the poor and tried to spread information about simple, useful remedies. He wanted to inform people about the many useful English herbs they could pick or buy cheaply — many people thought unusual foreign herbs were the only answer and they were often cheated by quacks. Culpeper became unpopular because of his Puritan sympathies, and suffered a chest wound fighting against the royalists in the Civil War.

The major remedies popularised during these years remained in use for a long time, occasionally supplemented by ideas from a new herbal. One such book called *Primitive Physic* was written by John Wesley who hoped to help members of his congregation who could not pay for professional treatment.

A further development occurred in 1790, when Samuel Hahnemann published a book on his homeopathic theories. This introduced many people to the idea of 'like cures like'. Remedies are prescribed which induce symptoms similar to those of the illness. Hahnemann regarded the symptoms of an illness as part of the body's defence and he aimed to strengthen that defence. Although the idea was not unknown to herbalists, it had not before been developed into a comprehensive theory.

During the nineteenth century, interest in herbalism declined. Modern medicine was rapidly gaining ground. Plant medicines were regarded as old-fashioned but they were not discarded: many modern drugs echo the chemistry of plants. Some muscle relaxants, for example, reflect the structure of curare — otherwise known as an arrow poison!

The twentieth century has gradually brought a change of attitude, and research into plant remedies has provided support for a variety of traditional uses. This has given rise to a new style of herbal, one of the first being *A Modern Herbal* by Mary Grieve (1931). With Hilda

Leyel, Mary Grieve also founded the *Herb Society*.

With interest in self-sufficiency during the sixties came books like Richard Mabey's *Food For Free*. This includes a section on herbs, advice on drinks such as dandelion coffee, and practical advice on finding and using safe plants.

More recent books illustrate the way in which modern herbal remedies have become accepted alongside other popular natural therapies. They include *The Natural Family Doctor* edited by Dr. Andrew Stanway. This gives advice on a range of therapies for those wanting to try self-help or those seeking professional advice.

Almost all the well-known herbals have been written by men, and this obscures an important fact — it was often women who administered the remedies, grew the plants, or ran the still-room. The role of women in this area, and the work they did, gave them an importance which is not often reflected in the books they used. One exception to this was *The English Housewife* by Gervase Markham (1615) — and it became a best-seller of its day. Modern books, like Kitty Little's *A Woman's Herbal* may be seen as descendants of this line.

Newspapers and magazines also reflect changing attitudes and information. One notable example of this concerned feverfew. Long used by herbalists to help migraine sufferers, research during the 1970s and 80s began supporting its use. Accounts in *The Lancet* and the *British Medical Journal* were followed by newspaper reports of feverfew's attributes. The *Daily Mail* told its readers of a 'Herbal way to weed out migraine', and the *Daily Telegraph* declared 'Herbal remedy better than latest cures'. *Titbits* called it a 'Wonder Weed' while *Woman's Realm* advised 'Grow Your Own Migraine Cure'. Feverfew is not the only herb under investigation. As further results are made known, more of the trial and error human testing of centuries may be supported by modern research.

Like various other medicinal herbs, feverfew grows easily and is suitable for most gardens. It is a popular choice with people who grow their own remedies. If you would like to grow some medicinal herbs, there are one or two things to keep in mind as you enjoy the pleasures of a living, growing medicine chest.

The plants and remedies suggested on the following pages are all for minor ailments. If you have a more serious disorder, it would be best to consult a professional herbalist. Also, there are various terms used in connection with herbal remedies which it is best to note from the start. In particular, *infusion* and *decoction* have precise meanings:

Infusion

An infusion is the method usually suggested when the leaves, flowers or stems of a plant are to be used. For a small amount, or single dose, use one teaspoon of dried herb (three teaspoons fresh) in a cup of water. Keep covered for about ten minutes. For larger amounts, add one ounce dried herb (three ounces fresh) to one pint of water.

It is possible to buy a herbal infuser from some suppliers. This a cup with a fitted strainer and lid.

Decoction

A decoction is usually suggested for woody herbs, or when the root is to be used. For one cup, or dose, use one teaspoon of the chopped, dried herb (three teaspoons fresh) to one cup of boiling water. Simmer gently for a few minutes, then strain. It is usually easier to make a larger amount using one ounce of dried herb (three ounces fresh) to 1½ pints of boiling water. Simmer gently for about 10-15 minutes, then strain.

If your remedy requires a plant that you have not yet grown, it is possible to buy various medical herbs packaged like tea in bags. You will find details of suppliers in Chapter 9.

Sleeplessness

As this can be related to tension or worry, it may be helpful to combine some method of relaxation, or a quiet occupation, with the chosen remedy.

Tea, coffee and cocoa do not help at bedtime as they are mild stimulants. A herbal tea can be much more helpful, particularly one such as lemon verbena (*Lippia citriodora*) or rosemary (*Rosmarinus officinalis*). Alternatively, you could make an infusion of camomile (*Chamaemelum nobile*) or hop flowers (*Humulus lupulus*). If you

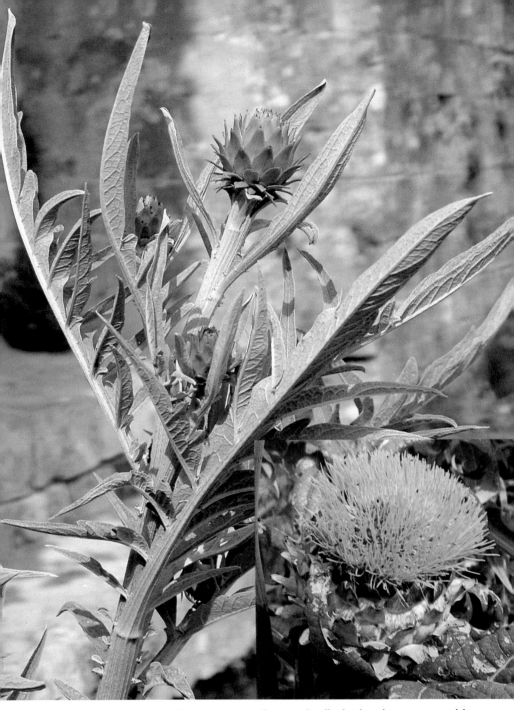

Artichoke leaves: an ingredient in tonics. Or, try the fleshy heads as a vegetable.

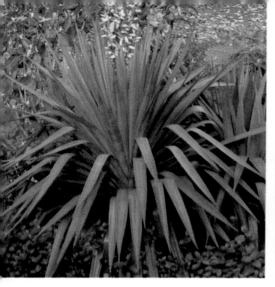
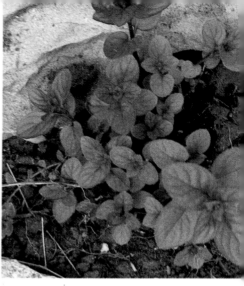

△ *Left*: *Aloe vera* leaves soothe sore skins. *Right*: Black peppermint tea for coughs and colds.

▽ Lesser celandine (*Ranunculus ficaria*), also known as pilewort. Traditionally used in ointment form to treat piles.

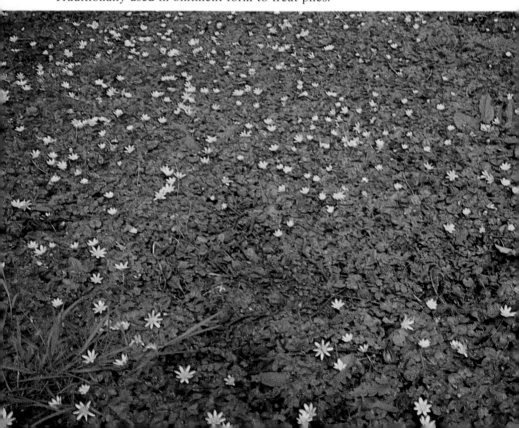

tend to wake during the night, keep some warm and ready for use. A thermos flask would do.

Other herbal aids include pillows filled with sleep-inducing flowers such as hops. Herbal baths can also help. Moderately hot water scented with lavender (*Lavandula officinalis*) or lime blossom (*Tilia europaea*) creates a gently relaxing mood-enhancer likely to aid sleep.

Colds and Coughs

Garlic (*Allium sativum*) is a traditional remedy for colds, particularly those leading to chest problems. Many people take garlic regularly to help prevent minor infections such as colds. If you enjoy the taste, you could chew several raw cloves. If not, garlic oil capsules or tablets could be taken. Garlic has been used medicinally since the time of the ancient Egyptians. It has many other internal and external uses in addition to its value against colds.

If you want to ease the symptoms of a cold, try an infusion of equal parts of elderflower (*Sambucus nigra*), peppermint (*Mentha piperita*) and hyssop (*Hyssopus officinalis*).

For a cough, where a remedy is required to bring up phlegm, a decoction of elecampane root (*Inula helenium*) is useful. If you are growing your own remedies, elecampane also happens to be a large, attractive plant.

Sore Throat

Red sage (*Salvia officinalis*) is often recommended as a gargle for sore throats. To make your own gargle: boil 4 ozs of fresh leaves in a mixture of ½ pint vinegar and ¾ pint water. Simmer for about 15 minutes, strain, cool, and bottle. Dilute to taste when required. A group of sage plants — red, green and golden — makes an attractive and useful addition to a herb garden.

Bleeding Gums

If you would like a mouthwash for this, try an infusion of mint leaves (*Mentha piperita*). It is also possible to buy herbal toothpaste. This usually includes echinacea or myrrh.

Headaches

The best-known herbal remedy for headaches is feverfew (*Tanacetum parthenium*, also known as *Chrysanthemum parthenium*). If you have your own plant, you can pick a fresh leaf and add it to salad or sandwiches. However, the taste is not too pleasant and you may prefer to make an infusion. There are also various traditional recipes in which wine, instead of water, is used for the infusion. If you dislike the taste of all these, feverfew tablets can be obtained from most health shops.

An alternative remedy is an infusion of lime flowers (*Tilia europaea*) but this is less highly regarded.

Migraine sufferers may also benefit from checking their diet as various foods such as tea, coffee, oranges, bananas and cheese are believed to trigger off attacks in some people.

Digestive Problems

An occasional decoction of dandelion root (*Taraxacum officinalis*) is a useful liver tonic.

Globe artichoke (*Cynara scolymus*) is also valued as a liver and kidney tonic. If you grow it, you have a beautiful plant with flower heads as a vegetable, and the leaves as a constituent of infusions.

Various herbs are considered aids to digestion. Marjoram (*Origanum marjorana*), for example, is used in food prepared for invalids as it increases the appetite.

Skin Care

Comfrey

This has been used as a herbal remedy for many years and can easily be grown in the garden. The main cultivated variety is Russian comfrey (*Symphytum perigrinum*). Crushed leaves can be applied in a poultice to sores and cuts, and the prepared ointment is useful for similar purposes and also for such things as bites and sunburn. The popularity of comfrey owes much to the work of Henry Doubleday, and products can be obtained from the Henry Doubleday Research Association (see Chapter 9 for details).

Aloe Juice

This soothes sore or irritated skin. It was so highly prized by the ancient Greeks — though they used it for a different purpose — that they were prepared to conquer the island of Socotra to obtain supplies. You could obtain supplies without any such difficulty. The plant (*Aloe vera*) grows well in this country, and the juice can be extracted by putting some clean, chopped leaves in a blender. Then strain off the juice.

Marigold

This is good for bruises. Make an infusion of the flowers (*Calendula officinalis*), and use the liquid to moisten a compress — then apply it to the affected area. A piece of clean lint can be used for the compress and bandaged into place.

Professional Herbalists

For general advice, or for more serious illnesses, you may want to consult a professional herbalist. If you do not know of one in your area, you can obtain the addresses of your nearest herbalists by writing to:

The National Institute of Medical Herbalists,
P. O. Box 3,
Winchester,
S022 6RR.

Herbalists are interested in treating the whole person, and prefer treatments which work gently and gradually. You may be surprised at the range of information a herbalist will find useful, and the many areas that treatment could cover. Alongside any suitable plant remedy, you may be asked to consider your diet, exercise, attitude to work, stress, or relationships. This is more likely to be necessary for a persistent problem but some minor ailments reflect other difficulties.

Generally speaking, herbalists prefer to use remedies made from the whole plant, while orthodox medicine usually tries to isolate and use particular substances or chemicals. Herbalists believe that as man and plants evolved together, plants have a unique role in healing.

A Garden of Herbs

The design and construction of a herb garden can be a rewarding experience, a source of great and growing pleasure. If you would enjoy a fragrant garden, or your own supply of fresh herbs, why not create a garden to meet your own requirements?

You might have a design in mind, or you might want to look at some of the designs that have proved successful over the years. Although few people have the opportunity to create designs on the scale of those at Villandry, for example, its knot gardens can still provide inspiration. Their clipped box hedges, creating a variety of symmetrical shapes, can be adapted to frame much smaller gardens. And the designs using flat geometric shapes filled with low-growing herbs can be reduced to suit many areas. Similarly, although few people have the resources to arrange large groups of medicinal herbs like those at Michelham Priory, the same principles of grouping according to use can be applied to herbs for your own reliable remedies. You might want a group for coughs and sore throats, or a group to soothe digestive problems.

Size is not particularly important. Many well-known gardens cover only a small area, and the scale of the most popular herbs is ideal for domestic gardens. You may not have Hatfield House as the backdrop to your garden but your chosen site may prove surprisingly rich and varied. For those with no outdoor space, window boxes and indoor gardens can still provide a good range of fresh herbs.

Outdoor Gardens

Whether you create or adapt a design, you will want it to reflect your own tastes and preferences. It should also maximise the advantages and minimise the disadvantages of your site. As the details emerge, you can then gradually decide what is to be kept,

95

moved, altered or bought. During the initial stages, you may want to keep various factors in mind:

The site

Some features of your site will be fixed starting-points. The size and perimeter of the land may be unchangeable but you could decide to use only part of the site if that would produce a better result. The distribution of even and uneven land might be helpful or some rearrangement may be necessary. As most herbs flourish in sunshine, it is useful to note any particularly sunny or shady areas.

The surroundings

Your site may adjoin a building. If so, some note should be taken of its style and shape. An informal garden might enhance a cottage, while a formal, geometric garden might be more suitable for a larger urban house. Some buildings have shapes or individual features that can be reflected in the garden design. Gables, unusual chimneys, window shapes, patterned brickwork, and so on, could provide a shape to be echoed in the design.

Open sites may have views that can also be incorporated into the design. This can give a pleasant feeling of depth and distance with selected herbs planted to provide a frame or contrast.

Enclosed sites are not necessarily less interesting. They may have walls, fences or trees which can be used to support or shelter herbs. Any long stretch of wall or fence could be broken by groups of tall free-standing herbs, or by wall-covering plants such as passion flower, some of the traditional roses, or fruits such as quince.

Style

In addition to considerations such as the style of the house and its surroundings, your design will need to be appropriate for the purpose of the garden. If, for example, you simply require a fragrant garden, access to individual plants will probably not be particularly important. But if you are growing herbs for culinary or medicinal uses, you will need to reach them with ease. Whatever your needs, the first stages of your design should show access. In a small garden, this could be as simple as a few carefully placed paving stones.

The access should be in keeping with the general style. Low beds of herbs surrounded by clipped box hedges would usually have pathways forming neat geometric shapes. An informal garden would be more likely to have less noticeable pathways, possibly partly hidden by plants.

Range of herbs

The range of herbs will be determined mainly by the purpose of the garden. However, even if your main interest is for example, culinary herbs, the plants can still be arranged in the way that proves most pleasing. The charts on pages 152 to 163 show such features as the colour, height and spread of the major herbs.

You might also be interested in ideas such as companion planting. Various combinations of plants tend to create beneficial effects and companion planting aims to make use of these pairings and groupings. For example, basil acts as an insect repellant and is useful near tomatoes. Chives are thought to prevent black spot on roses, and various plants such as nasturtium and sage are disliked by many pests and prove useful to general garden health.

It is also useful to note which plants are annual, biennial, or perennial. And some plants have particular features that may require attention. For example, mints may need to be planted within a hidden container to control spreading.

Accessories

Traditional herb gardens had a distinctive range of accessories, particularly for use at the heart of the design. Sundials, bird-baths, statues and fountains have all been used for this purpose. Other features are typical of a particular period. Turf benches and heraldic ornaments were popular in Tudor gardens, temples and busts were more popular in the eighteenth century.

As an alternative to garden ornaments, certain trees could be introduced into the design. Trees such as juniper, witch hazel, barberry and fig would be useful as well as attractive.

A Sample Design For A Small Herb Garden

The garden shown in plan 1, and in the photographs on pages 99 and 100, was developed in an abandoned sunken garden.

Plan 1

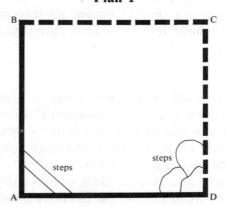

Site

The site is quite well-drained, situated about halfway down a long sloping lawn which has been grassed for some years.

Sides AB and AD have stone walls. Sides BC and CD are grass slopes. The steps at 'A' are in good condition, those at 'D' are not. There are currant bushes along AB, an elder bush and greater periwinkle along BC. There is a rose bush below an apple tree alongside CD. The area towards CD is shadier than the area towards AB.

The surroundings

One end of the lawn adjoins the owner's modern stone house. The other end is separated from farmland and several good oak trees by a low wooden fence.

Style

It was decided to retain the square shape of the garden, to mend the steps at D, and to provide access to the herbs by adding further stones to the base. The garden will most often be entered from 'A', so taller herbs (except those requiring most sunshine) were introduced into the area shown shaded on plan 2. In addition, honeysuckle has been planted against the bare areas of fence.

The simple shape of the garden with its background of stone walls and grassy slopes is in keeping with the general style of the garden, also with the house which has a stone-paved patio where more herbs are grown.

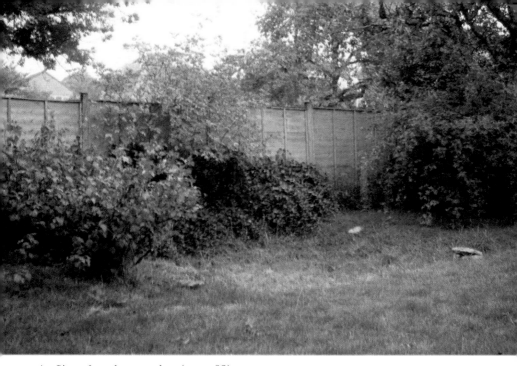

△ Site of sunken garden (page 98).

▽ Clearing area around sunken garden.

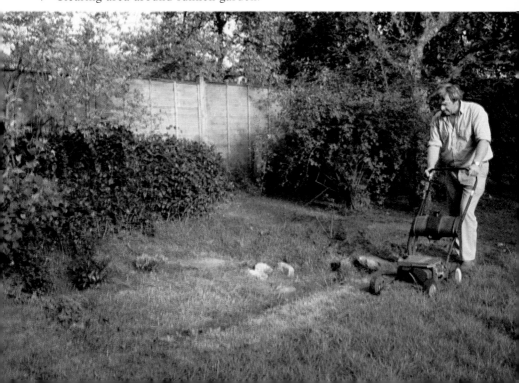

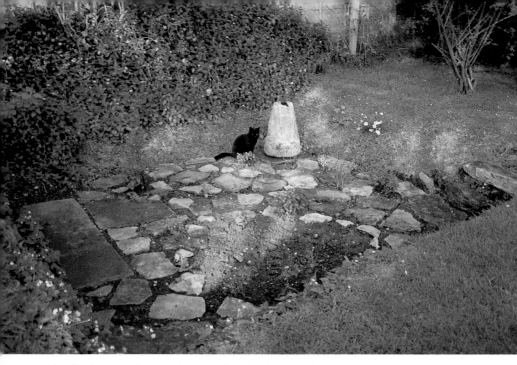

△ Sunken garden partly completed, with the first plants in place.

▽ Sunken herb garden after the first six months.

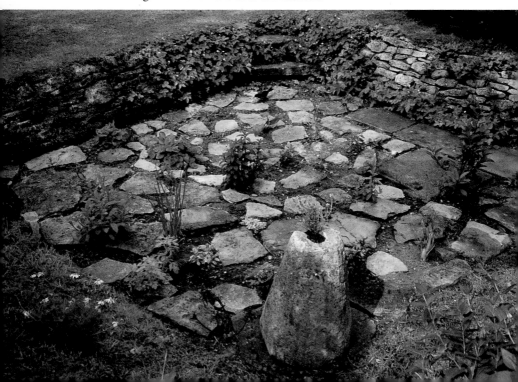

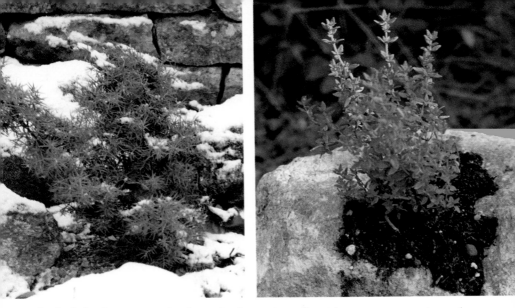

△ *Left*: Juniper, attractive in rockeries and small outdoor arrangements, and as bonsai plants indoors. *Right*: Thyme growing in the hollow top of a stone ornament.

▽ Jasmine, a scented background plant for the patio.

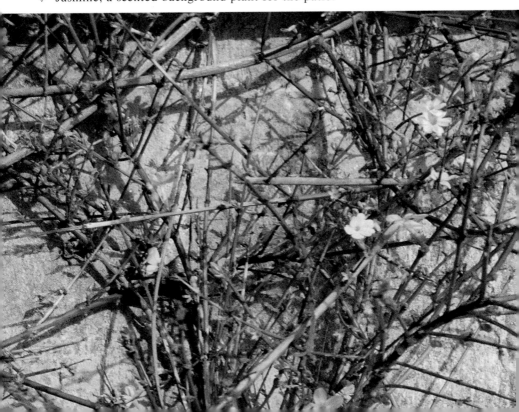

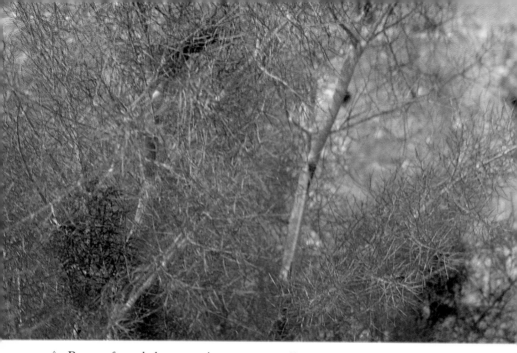

△ Bronze fennel shown against a stone wall.

▽ Lily-of-the-valley, a fragrant herb — plant near a window, doorway or garden seat.

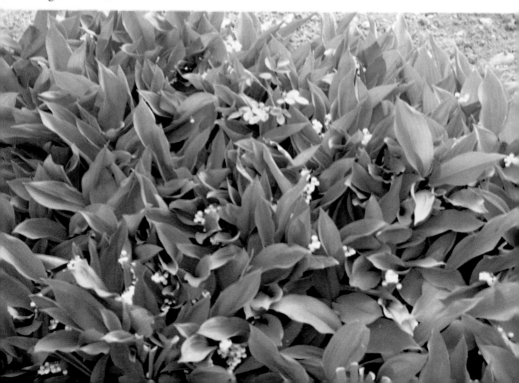

Plan 2

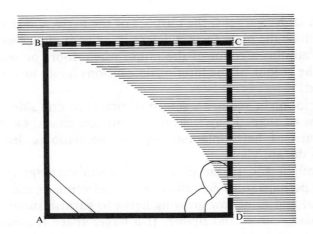

Range of herbs

The main requirement was a garden of culinary herbs with some additional herbs for medicinal or decorative purposes. The taller plants include bay (*Laurus nobilis*), fennel (*Foeniculum vulgare*), rosemary (*Rosmarinus officinalis*), and lovage (*Levisticum officinale*). The greater periwinkle (*Vince major*) has been left to cover part of the slope along BC. The slope CD has been left grassed but various plants have been added such as mint (*Mentha piperita*), thyme (*Thymus vulgaris*), and marjoram (*Origanum vulgare*). These will be left to grow and flower on the grassy slope.

Wild strawberries were already growing in the cracks of the stone walls. These have been left untouched, and here and there other plants have been added such as thyme (*Thymus Doone Valley*).

Accessories

The sunken, slightly secret appearance of the garden has been retained. One ornamental stone has been introduced to provide a feature at 'C'. This has a hollow top in which thyme (*Thymus vulgaris*) is growing.

The photographs on page 100 show the gradual progress of the garden as further herbs were introduced and more stone was added to provide access.

Patios

As with larger gardens, the purpose of the herbs and the nature of the site will be the main factors determining your choice of plants. If the patio adjoins a room of the house when doors or windows are opened, the colour of the interior decorations might also need to be considered.

The patio might require a screen of plants to one side, perhaps a simple row of shaped bay trees in elegant containers. Or you might want groups of herbs planted beyond the patio to lead the eye towards a distant view.

Herbs might add to the pleasure of warm evenings entertaining friends — perhaps some containers with a selection of mint for juleps or Pimm's, and some low-growing herbs to garnish summer snacks: parsley, basil, chives and thyme. If a larger space is available, you could create an interesting decorative effect by introducing some of the herbs with cocktail connections: vervain (*Verbena officinalis*), the herb that flavours vermouth; juniper (*Juniperus communis*) with the berries that flavour gin; angelica (*Angelica archangelica*) used in Benedictine; and sweet woodruff (*Asperula odorata*), a dainty herb used in wines.

If your patio includes a barbecue, you could grow a plant such as sweet peppers (*Capsicum annuum*). These will grow and ripen if they are in a very sheltered position or if your patio has an adjoining glassed area. French tarragon (*Artemisia dracunculus*) is useful to add to barbecued chicken.

Where the patio adjoins the house, or if you have a pergola or trellis nearby, a scented background plant such as honeysuckle, jasmine or an old-fashioned rose might provide an additional feature.

Window-boxes

If you are preparing window boxes, they may be part of your total garden design, or they may be the only place you have available to grow outdoor plants. In either case, you will want to consider various points before you buy plants.

How do the window boxes relate to the rest of your garden design?

Will the colour and height of the plants, and the style of the window-boxes, suit the building?

If you are growing culinary herbs, can you reach them easily?

If you are growing fragrant herbs, are they near a window that is often open, or near a garden seat or doorway?

When you are satisfied with these aspects of your design, the boxes for the herbs should be at least 20 centimeters deep, with a thin layer of drainage material at the base and compost above. Although smaller herbs such as parsley, chives, thyme and marjoram will be most suitable, slightly larger ones such as rosemary, sage and tarragon can be clipped to the desired height. With rosemary, it is also possible to grow the prostrate variety and this can create a pleasant 'cascade' effect. The smaller varieties of juniper and lavender would also be suitable. Window-boxes in very sheltered positions could also include delicate plants such as basil or peppers.

If you are growing herbs particularly for their fragrance, pinks, lily-of-the-valley or violet are good choices. There are also various attractive small herbs which benefit from being seen at close quarters: wild pansy, pasque flower, wood sorrel, or sweet woodruff.

Although most herbs have small or subtly-coloured flowers, it is always worthwhile to check the exact colour if you have bought the plant before flowering or have grown it from seed. Interesting and colourful effects can be created by choosing plants with variegated or unusual-coloured leaves. Sage is particularly rich in leaf types.

Indoor Gardens

A large variety of containers is now available for indoor gardens. These come in many sizes, shapes and levels. Whether you want an indoor herb garden for its usefulness or its beauty, a suitable container in a suitable position is a must. Unlike some plants grown indoors, nearly all herbs love sunshine so an area with some direct sunlight is best.

If you are growing herbs for use in the kitchen, you might like to grow them alongside other edible plants. Aubergine (*Solanum melongena ovigerum*) will grow successfully indoors and can be kept to a height of about 30 centimeters. There are also several tomato varieties such as Tiny Tim which would be suitable. Marigold and nasturtium are useful for salads and will add colour to a mixture of plants such as parsley and cress.

If you are growing herbs indoors for decorative purposes, there are many possibilities. Although juniper is one of the most popular herbs in small outdoor arrangements and rockeries, it is also often used indoors as a bonsai plant. It could form part of a decorative arrangement, possibly with a pine-scented pot-pourri, or it could grow alongside other herbs with woody stems.

Alternatively you might want an arrangement that would reflect the style of a traditional outdoor herb garden. This could be achieved using miniature roses (usually 15-30 centimeters in height) as a background, while concentrating on small-leaved herbs such as thyme for the foreground.

If you prefer something similar to the usual range of indoor plants, a bowl of saffron crocus (*Crocus sativus*) could be grown alongside bowls of other spring bulbs. On a larger scale, a medicine plant (*Aloe vera*) could be grown with other succulents such as the larger Echiverias.

Selecting your herbs

The beauty of most herbs comes from their shape, scent and leaves. In some cases such as passion flower or roses, the flower may be the focus of attention. In traditional herb gardens, it was the ornamental combination of these attributes, and their symbolic meaning, which gave each pathway or corner its distinctive character. We may no longer believe that the flowers of skullcap (*Scutellaria lateriflora*) look like little helmets to show us its medicinal value (for headaches or insomnia) but like mandrake or bloodroot, its image lingers. A modern garden which includes some of the herbs known and used for centuries can provide a glimpse of the past alongside its other pleasures.

The charts on the following pages give brief details of some of the most popular herbs. You may want to check such things as height or flower colour before adding a plant to your garden.

A View of Herbs

It is still possible to see the original designs of a few early herb gardens. Some have remained relatively undisturbed; others have been restored or changed to suit modern tastes. If you are working on your own herb garden, you may want to develop an individual design, or you may want to adapt one of the classic or modern layouts seen in gardens open to the public. The important thing to remember is that designs can be rearranged to suit different sites, scales and surroundings.

It is thought that the early herb garden designs were inspired by the Arab patterns introduced into this country by sailors and other travellers. The intricate geometric shapes worked best with ground-hugging plants able to provide a range of colours. Before long, various changes and elaborations came into fashion, and the appropriately-named 'knot garden' became a popular feature of fashionable gardens in the sixteenth and seventeenth centuries.

John Parkinson, the king's herbalist, described the art of planting kont gardens in his book, *Paradise in Sole Paradisus Terrestris* (1629):

You may first observe the several kinds of (plant) that do flower at one and the same time, and then place them in such order and so near one to another, that their flowers appearing together of several colours, will cause the more admiration in beholders, thus: the vernal crocus or saffron flowers of the spring, white, purple, yellow and striped, with some vernal colchicum ·or meadow saffron among them; some Dens Canis or dog's teeth, and some of the small early leucojum or bulbous violet, all planted in some proportion as near to one another as is fit for them, will give such grace to the garden, that the place will seem like a piece of tapestry of many glorious colours, to increase everyone's delight.

One of Parkinson's own designs at Thornham Magna in Suffolk suffered a period of neglect but there are plans for its restoration. Modern examples of the style can be seen at Pollock House in Glasgow, The Tudor House Museum in Southampton, and at Hatfield House in Hertfordshire. Typically, the design had a central statue, sundial or tree and the pattern radiated from it. At Southampton, the garden was devised during 'The Year Of The Garden' (1979) to replace the one lost after Sir Richard Lister had inhabited the house during the reign of Henry VIII. The current design has a central knot garden surrounded by four raised herb beds. A pergola, arbour and secret garden are also included in the design. Generally, Tudor gardens featured turf seats and these may also be added. They were brick benches about eighteen inches high which were then covered with turf to create a more natural appearance. They provided a place to appreciate the garden at leisure and possibly observe such features as those described in *A Midsummer Night's Dream*:

I know a bank where the wild thyme blows,
Where oxlips and the nodding violet grows
Quite over-canopied with luscious woodbine,
With sweet musk-roses, and with eglantine. . .

The 'eglantine' of Shakespeare and Chaucer's time is known to us as the sweet briar rose (*Rosa rubiginosa*). It is still occasionally seen in old gardens and hedgerows particularly on chalky soil in the south of England.

Although knot gardens were typical of the period and fashionable, they did have their critics. Francis Bacon commented that they were '. . . but toys; you may see as good sights many times in tarts'. However, his description of what he would prefer sounds much the same to modern gardeners: '. . . little low hedges round like welts, with some pretty pyramids.'

As time passed, new fashions emerged but at first they differed little from the knot garden. The parterre, though usually on a grander scale, was still a very formal design, something like a very large and intricate carpet of plants, close to the ground and best seen from one of the high windows in the grand house to be found nearby. Like the knot garden, the parterre dates from the classic years of herb gardening when the books of Gerard, Culpeper and Parkinson were in use.

These gardens, like their predecessors, were not universally admired. Alexander Pope commented:

On every side you look, behold the wall!
No pleasing intricacies intervene,
No artful wildness to perplex the scene:
Grove nods at grove, each alley has a brother,
And half the platform just reflects the other.

But most people found the new style acceptable. It was a formal garden for a formal age. Restorations of these elegant gardens can be seen at Little Moreton Hall, Hosely Old Hall and Ham House. The National Trust of Scotland has also recreated a parterre at Pitmedden.

As tastes changed and less formal gardens were planted, herbs escaped from the rigid patterns of the past. From these years of 'informal' designs, many of the most attractive herb gardens to have survived are the ones that formed part of the kitchen gardens beside large farmhouses or manor houses. A good example can be seen at Cogges Manor Farm in Oxfordshire. Here, the herbs grow alongside a traditional selection of fruit and vegetables. There is no formal design — except the use of a lavender hedge — but there are many attractive effects created by colour contrasts and the background of mellow stone walls. It is also possible to see some of the herbs drying naturally above the range in the nearby farm kitchen.

Such gardens occurred on a smaller scale beside some cottages. They are described by Flora Thompson in *Lark Rise to Candleford*:

The men took great pride in their gardens and allotments and there was always competition amongst them as to who should have the earliest and choicest of each kind. Fat green peas, broad beans as big as a halfpenny, cauliflowers a child could make an armchair of, runner beans and cabbage and kale, all in their seasons went into the pot with the roly-poly and strip of bacon.

Then they ate plenty of green food, all home-grown and freshly pulled; lettuce and radishes and young onions with pearly heads and leaves like fine grass. A few slices of bread and home-made lard, flavoured with rosemary . . .

Gradually, the design of herb-gardens became more varied and a wider range of styles became acceptable both for larger and smaller sites. In some cases, sensitive restorations produced interesting gardens on sites abandoned for many years. At Beaulieu Abbey, for example, the monks' original garden was established during the Middle Ages but its design was overgrown and lost. During recent years, a new garden using traditional plants has been planted. It includes many of the most popular herbs, also such plants as stinking hellebore and comfrey which are seen less often.

At Knebworth House in Hertfordshire, the herb garden is based on designs by Gertrude Jekyll. Here the herb gardens are edged with brick which provides a warm colour-contrast with the herbs. A brick wall and statues give shelter and echo the designs of earlier times.

A less usual site for a herb garden is found in the grounds of Castle Drogo, built for Julius Drewe by Sir Edwin Lutyens. The house was completed in 1930 and is a blend of modern design and ancient stronghold high above the Teign Gorge on the eastern slopes of Dartmoor. The herb garden forms part of the image the house seeks.

Herbs can also be seen at various botanical gardens. In some cases, these are of interest chiefly because of the range of plants; in other cases, various features of the layout may be the point of attraction. The Chelsea Physic Garden, for example, has the earliest known rock garden in this country. It was created from basaltic lava brought from Iceland by Sir Joseph Banks in 1772. The garden was established in 1673 by the Society of Apothecaries, and has a long history of research into the medicinal uses of plants. Today, it provides facilities for studies by various colleges of the University of London. King's College, for example, grows feverfew in order to investigate its use as a treatment for migraine. The garden also conducts some research of its own; recently this concerned sages.

Before the Embankment was built in 1874, the garden was reached by boat, and some plants and trees actually arrived by river. The rich riverside soil and sheltered position encouraged the growth of many plants which would not otherwise be seen in the city. At one time, only those with a professional interest in plants could visit the garden but during the last decade it has been opened to the public.

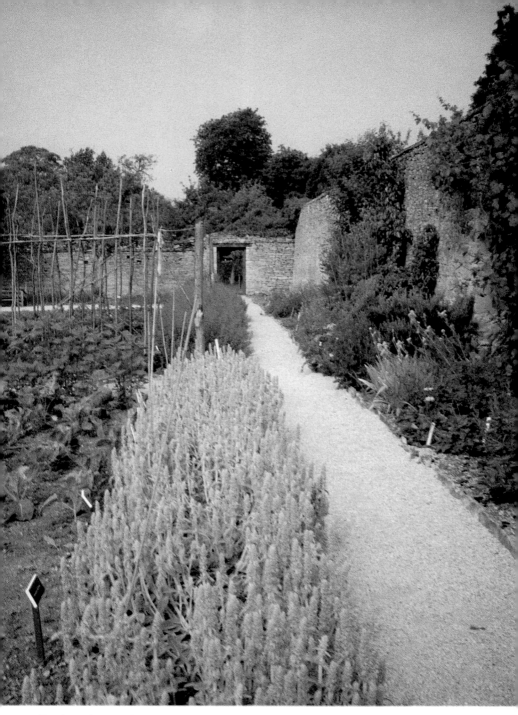

Garden, Cogges Manor Farm.

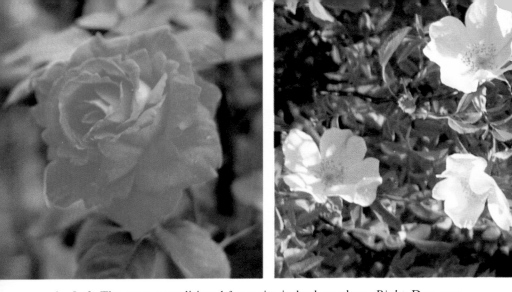

△ *Left*: The rose, a traditional favourite in herb gardens. *Right*: Dog rose.

▽ Passion flower, an evocation of Christ's Passion, and grown in herb gardens connected with an abbey or priory.

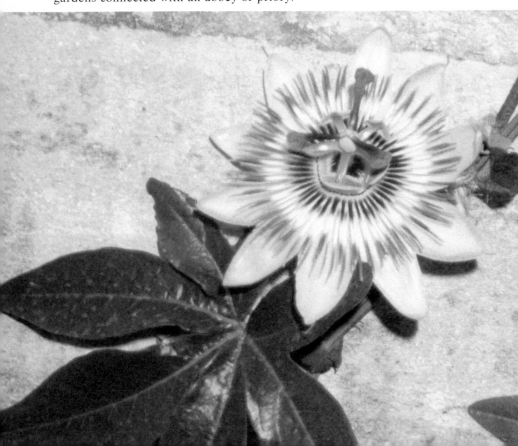

The Royal Botanic Gardens at Kew are of interest for several reasons. There are some notable layouts including the traditional one in Queen Anne's Garden. And since 1983, the Pharmaceutical Society's *Collection of Crude Drugs and Herbaria* has been housed in the Herbarium Library. The Gardens, in collaboration with the publishers Century, have produced a book about the collection. It is called *Nature's Pharmacy* and provides an account of major items from the collection and their place in the development of 'green medicine'. The story stretches back in time to evidence that Stone Age man suffered from arthritis and used various plants to treat this and other conditions. One of the plants thought to have been used was hollyhock which has long been known as the 'poor man's aspirin'. Various well-known plant products are discussed — curare and digitalis, for example — and also the current interest in various plant drugs and the fact that many synthetic drugs mimic natural plant structures.

Although botanic gardens in other parts of the country are smaller than those at Kew, they often devote some space to herbs. The Oxford Botanical Garden uses herbs in rockeries round the lily pond. These include various junipers and thymes, which provide a range of silver, green and blue tones amongst the rocks. There are also various small arrangements of herbs in old stone pots beside the house, and a rose garden planted to an unusual design.

Other herb gardens have developed associations with particular people or illustrate particular themes. There are herb gardens in Stratford-Upon-Avon at Anne Hathaway's cottage and Shakespeare's birthplace where you can see many of the herbs popular during Elizabethan times and recall some of their old names and uses.

In *The Merry Wives of Windsor* Mistress Anne Page wants the elves to get busy with the cleaning:

The several chairs of order look you scour
With juice of balm, and every precious flower.

In *King Lear* a scene is set with descriptions of plants nearby:

Crown'd with rank fumiter and furrow-weeds,
With burdocks, hemlocks, nettles, cuckoo-flowers.

Another garden with literary associations is at Burwash in Sussex, once the home of Rudyard Kipling. Here we can see some of the plants and scenes that inspired memorable evocations of rural England. Adults may think of the poems, while children may think of Puck and his talks to Dan and Una. He introduces them to the old ways, to the plants and trees and people who embody the spirit of the past.

One plant common to most old herb gardens was the rose. The traditional varieties can be seen at Mottisfont in Hampshire where the National Trust has developed a superb collection. Roses have remained popular and there are now about 10,000 varieties. These include the traditional ones as well as those of particular value for medicine or cosmetics. The traditional apothecary's rose (*Rosa gallica officinalis*) is having something of a revival with the current interest in aromatherapy.

Possibly the best-known traditional rose is the 'dog rose' (*Rosa canina*). The reasons given for its name tend to vary. Some argue that its name refers to its use as a cure for rabies. Others favour the idea that its thorns look like daggers. This caused it to become known as the 'dag rose' but the name was corrupted to 'dog rose'.

The rose is also rich in other historical associations. 'Celestial' was the favourite rose of Henry VIII and was grown at Hampton Court Palace where many features of the Tudor gardens can still be seen. The Wars of the Roses gave rise to many well-known associations for red and white roses. The 'queen of flowers' has a long history in other countries too, and in the United States, there are fossil remains of roses believed to be 35 million years old.

Alongside the rose petals in a traditional pot-pourri, you will usually find some lavender heads. Although it cannot claim as many varieties as the rose, this is another plant which has remained very popular. If you wish to find out more about it, Norfolk Lavender would be a good place to visit. Although the plant is usually grown for its beauty or scent, it can also be used in cooking. Recipes such as rabbit with lavender make a pleasant change from the more usual combinations of meat and herbs.

Some gardens have been planted to illustrate quite different themes. At Michelham Priory in Sussex, the plants are grouped according to their uses. One group is useful for wounds and broken bones, and includes plants such as comfrey (which used to be known as 'knitbone'). Another group is for heart, lung or blood problems. And a separate section has plants for household uses. If you are interested in plants for these purposes, it can be rewarding to see them grouped in this way.

The Michelham Priory garden has been laid out quite recently but it reflects a long tradition. Herb gardens were often connected with religious buildings and many of the beliefs surrounding herbs reflect their use by monks and nuns. Angelica, for example, was believed to have been given its name by a monk after an angel revealed its use as a cure for the plague. Passion flower is probably the best-known example with its evocation of Christ's Passion: the corolla represents the crown of thorns, the styles are the nails, the stamens the hammer, the pointed leaves the spear, and the tendrils the whip. It is worthwhile to bear these connections in mind, and if you are visiting an abbey or priory look for any herbs nearby.

If your interest in herbs is part of a general interest in gardening, you could visit the National Centre for Organic Gardening at Ryton-on-Dunsmore. Here you will find a herb and rose garden alongside a wild flower meadow, pond, and conservation area. The garden is run by the Henry Doubleday Association which has promoted organic gardening for many years. It was founded by Henry Doubleday (1813-1902), a quaker smallholder who was particularly interested in the use of comfrey. Today, the plant is popular with organic gardeners as a compost activator. It also has various medicinal uses and is rich in vitamins, minerals and trace elements. Unfortunately, it is not particularly appetising and this is probably why it did not become as popular for culinary use as Doubleday had hoped.

Interesting herb gardens are open to the public. If you would enjoy a garden visit organised with lectures and other information, you can obtain details from:

The Herb Society,
77 Great Peter Street,
London SW1 (01-222-3634).

Many of our larger private gardens also include herbs, and although these may not be open on a regular year-round basis, they can often be visited as part of the National Gardens Scheme. This started in 1927, when 600 gardens opened during the year. There are now large numbers of gardens open throughout the country and details can be obtained from:

The National Gardens Scheme,
57 Lower Belgrave Street,
London SW1W 0LR.

The wide range of herb gardens open to the public should not obscure the fact that many herbs can be found growing wild throughout Britain. In my own area, there is a disused quarry, visited by few people, where many wild flowers and herbs have found a home. Water mint grows beside a stretch of water on the quarry floor with a carpet of wild strawberries on the surrounding dry areas. On the steep banks at the side, there are spotted heath orchids with dog rose and sweet briar above. One stony area has been colonised by elder and hemlock, another by valerian. The quarry covers several acres and a walk in almost any direction will reveal more plants.

As with all wild plants, herbs should be left growing untouched. However, if you are offered a sprig from a cultivated plant, or buy one, remember the language of flowers: a sprig of rosemary symbolises remembrance but basil (known as kiss-me-Nicholas in parts of Italy) means that lovers need not keep their distance! (see Chapter 1).

Some Addresses

Abbey House Museum, Abbey Road, Kirkstall, Leeds. Telephone: (0532) 755821.

Acorn Bank, Temple Sowerby, Cumbria. Telephone: Sue Ryder Home, Chris Braithwaite (0930) 61281.

The American Museum in Britain, Claverton Manor, Bath, Avon. Telephone: (0225) 60503

Anne Hathaway's Cottage, Shottery, Stratford-Upon-Avon, Warwickshire.

Barnsley House Gardens, Barnsley, Cirencester, Gloucestershire. (Open Monday-Friday, 10 am-6 pm).

Bateman's (home of Rudyard Kipling), Burwash, Etchingham, East Sussex. Telephone: (0435) 882302.

Beaulieu Palace House and Gardens, Beaulieu, Brockenhurst, Hampshire, Telephone: (0590) 612345.

Cambridge University Botanic Garden, Cambridge (gates in Trumpington Road, Hills Road and Bateman Street). Telephone: (0223) 337733.

Cogges Manor Farm Museum, Witney, Oxfordshire. Telephone: (0993) 72602.

Candlesby Herbs, Cross Keys, Spilsby, Lincolnshire. Telephone: (075 485) 211.

Castle Drogo, near Chagford, Newton Abbot, Devon. Telephone: (064 73) 3306.

Chelsea Physic Garden, 66 Royal Hospital Road, London SW3. Telephone: (01)352 5646.

Curtis Museum, Allen Gallery, Church Street, High Street, Alton, Hampshire. Telephone: (0420) 82802.

The Country Demonstration Garden, Probus (Nr. Truro) Cornwall.

Dartington Hall, near Totnes, Devon, Telephone: (0803) 862224.

East Lambrook Manor, South Petherton, Somerset. Telephone: (0460) 40328.

Eyhorne Manor, Hollingbourne, Maidstone, Kent. Telephone: (062 780) 514.

Felbrigg Hall, near Cromer, Norfolk. Telephone: (026 375) 444.

Gunby Hall, near Spilsby, Lincolnshire.

Hardwick Hall, Chesterfield, Derbyshire. Telephone: (0246) 850430.

Hampton Court Palace, East Molesey, Surrey.

Hatfield House, Hatfield, Hertfordshire. Telephone: (070 72) 62823.

Herterton House, Hartington, Cambo, Morpeth, Northumberland. (Closed Tuesday and Thursday.) Telephone: (067 074) 278.

Hever Castle, Edenbridge, Kent.

Hidcote Manor Garden, Hidcote Bartrim, Chipping Campden, Gloucestershire. Telephone: (0386 438) 333.

Knebworth House, Knebworth, Hertfordshire. Telephone: (0438) 812661.

Little Moreton Hall, Congleton, Cheshire. Telephone: (026 02) 2018.

University of Liverpool Botanic Gardens, Neston, South Wirral.

Michelham Priory, Upper Dicker, Hailsham, East Sussex. Telephone: (0323) 844224.

Moseley Old Hall, Fordhouses, Wolverhampton, West Midlands. (Open weekends until end June: Wednesday-Sunday through summer.) A knot garden with a parterre being planted. Telephone: (0902) 782808.

Mottisfont, Nr. Romsey, Hampshire. (National Trust collection of traditional roses.)

National Centre For Organic Gardening, Ryton-On-Dunsmore, Coventry. Telephone: (0203) 303517.

Norfolk Lavender Limited, Caley Mill, Heacham, King's Lynn, Norfolk. Telephone: (0485) 70384.

Oxford Botanic Garden, High Street, Oxford. Telephone: (0865) 242.

Pitmedden House, nr. Oldmeldrum, Formartine, Scotland.

Priorwood Garden, Melrose, Roxburghshire. Telephone: (089 682) 2555.

Red House Museum, Quay Road, Christchurch, Dorset. Telephone: (0202) 482860.

The Royal Botanic Gardens, Kew, Surrey. Telephone: (01) 940 1171.

RHS Gardens, Wisley, Woking, Surrey. Telephone: (0483) 224234.

Shakespeare's Birthplace, Henley Street, Stratford-Upon-Avon, Warwickshire.

Sissinghurst Castle Garden, Sissinghurst, Cranbrook, Kent. Telephone: (0580) 712850.

Tudor House Museum, Bugle Street, Southampton, Hampshire. Telephone: (0703) 24216.

Welsh Folk Museum, St. Fagans, Cardiff. Telephone: (0222) 569441.

A Purchase of Herbs

Many of the items you are likely to require can be bought locally from shops or garden centres. But there are certain specialist plants and preparations that you may need to obtain from outside your area. The addresses in this chapter are organised to aid your search.

Some of the companies and organisations listed have interesting histories that reflect changing attitudes to herbs and their uses. Culpepers, and the Henry Doubleday Research Association, for example, were founded by people who wanted to supply information and materials to those who shared their views. The growth of their organisations, particularly in recent years, shows how demand for their products has risen. Further details can be found below the addresses.

Some suppliers close down and others start up, so you may find it useful to keep an additional list of your own. Also, each person has his own particular interest: culinary herbs, essential oils for aromatherapy, equipment for infusions, and so on. For this reason, you might want to extend one particular area of the list.

Plants and Seeds

Wells and Winter,
Mere House,
Near Maidstone,
Kent.

Provide a mail order service offering herb and wildflower seeds, also herb plants and small-scale garden equipment. The seeds cover a good standard selection. The plants include some less usual varieties: eleven types of mint, five varieties of sage, several varieties of lavender and thyme.

There is an auction of surplus plants on the last Saturday of

September each year, and copies of *A Herb Grower's Notebook* can also be purchased. The delivery service is carefully organised. When we ordered some plants near Christmas, we were told that they would be delivered but not by post as the plants might suffer from Christmas delays. Sir Peter Wells happened to be going to a function near our home, so he dropped the plants off on the way. It was the first time we had met a knighted 'delivery man'.

Suffolk Herbs Ltd.,
Sawyers Farm,
Little Cornard,
Sudbury,
Suffolk, C010 0NY
Tel: 0787 227247

They supply a wide range of seeds by post, particularly herbs and wild flowers as well as seeds for specialist interests such as oriental vegetables. Their mail order service includes various dried herbs and spices, also books on herbs and related subjects. There is a comprehensive, descriptive catalogue.

Suttons Seeds Ltd.,
Hele Road,
Torquay,
Devon. TQZ 7QJ
Tel: 0803 612011

Offer a selection of the most popular herbs, including two types of fennel and two types of marjoram. Also a good range of vegetables and various items such as mung beans to suit particular recipes or tastes.

John Chambers,
15 Westleigh Road,
Barton Seagrave,
Kettering,
Northamptonshire NN15 5AL
Tel: 0933 681632

John Chambers is best known as a supplier of wildflower seeds, bulbs and plants. He also supplies seeds for herbs and some 'edible plants', with appropriate books and wallcharts if required. The wildflower seeds come in many groups: for woodlands and wetlands, clay and lime, hedgerows and meadows. The herb seed collections include culinary, medicinal, dyeing and unusual 'best selling' herbs. There is also a collection of seeds for alternative food plants.

The catalogue provides quite detailed information about each plant or seed type. There is also some useful general information about wildflowers and herbs.

Hollington Nurseries Ltd,
Woolton Hill,
Newbury,
Berks. RG15 9XT
Tel: 0635 253908

Although Hollington Nurseries sell a range of plants, herbs form a major part of their sales. They supply herb seeds by mail order and herb plants from the site. The staff also provide advice on herb-garden design. Two publications about herbs are available, a *Herb Manual* and *Herbs*, the latter being a guide to herbs as garden plants. Old-fashioned roses, scented shrubs and trees can also be purchased.

Trevor White,
'Old Fashioned Roses'
24 White Hart Street,
Aylsham,
Norfolk, NR11 6HG
Tel: 0263 734975

Plants can be bought by mail order or by visiting the site. Some modern roses are available but the bulk of the plants are varieties from old-fashioned groups such as Albas, Gallicas, Damasks and Bourbons.

Iden Croft Herbs,
Frittenden Road,
Staplehurst,
Kent.
Tel: 0580 891432

Will supply some plants by post — contact for details.

Heches Herbs,
St. Peter in the Wold,
Channel Islands.
Tel: 0 481 63345
They provide a mail order service and will send a herb list on request.

Oak Cottage Herb Farm,
Nesscliffe,
Near Shrewsbury
Shropshire.
Tel: 074381 262
Will supply by post.

Herbs and Herb Products from Organic Suppliers

Ryton Gardens,
The National Centre For Organic Gardening,
Ryton-On-Dunsmore,
Coventry,
CV8 3LG

Ryton Gardens is concerned with organic gardening in general and herb seeds can be purchased. They are listed in the catalogue with details of their growth and use. A herb garden has been designed as part of the displays.

If you want an organic herb garden this would be an ideal place to visit. You can examine organic fertilisers, compost makers, techniques of pest and disease control without chemicals. To complete your day, a good range of books and organic wines is available.

The gardens are run by the Henry Doubleday Research Association. If you are likely to have a long-term interest in organic gardening, this would be a suitable association to join. Many people became interested following the TV series 'All Muck and Magic!' which showed the work of the association and ways in which domestic gardens could follow organic methods. The booklet for the series provides a good, brief guide to organic gardening.

The association is well-known for encouraging the use of comfrey.

Some comfrey products can be obtained at the gardens, others are available from Herbal Laboratories.

Another address you might find useful is:

The Organic Growers Association,
86-88 Colston Street,
Bristol BS1 5BB
Tel: 0272 299666/299800

An associated organisation is:

The Soil Association,
86-88 Colston Street,
Bristol, BS1 5BB
Tel: 0272 290661

General Herbal Products and Preparations

Culpeper

Culpeper was founded in 1927 by Mrs. C.F. Leyel, and now has many branches. It takes its name from the great herbalist Nicholas Culpeper (1616-1652) who ran his practice from Red Lion Street, Spitalfields, in London. He wanted herbs and herbal remedies to be widely available, particularly to the poor. His book *The Complete Herbal* was published in 1649.

Culpeper shops sell herbal products produced in natural ways. They avoid testing on animals and using contentious animal products. Their mail order list can be obtained from their head office or from your nearest branch.

Mrs Leyel was also one of the two founders of the Herb Society which retains an interest in Culpeper. Her partner in establishing the Herb Society was Mary Grieve, whose book *A Modern Herbal* (first published in 1931) is still popular. Mary Grieve ran a herb nursery at Chalfont St. Peter where she grew many medicinal herbs. They proved particularly useful during the drug shortages of the First World War. Her experiences during those years encourage her to write her book and to advocate the wider use of herbs.

Head Office,
Culpeper Shops,
Hadstock Road,
Linton,
Cambridge CB1 6NJ
Tel: 1223 891196

Gerard House

Like Culpeper, Gerard House is named after a famous herbalist. In this case it is John Gerard, author of the *Herball*.

Their mail order service provides quite a wide range of products: herbal preparations, dietary supplements, ointments, biochemic tissue salts, herbal teas, cosmetics and essential oils. There are also certain remedies developed by Gerard House for specific purposes.

Gerard House,
3 Wickham Road,
Boscombe,
Bournmouth,
Dorset BH7 6JX
Tel: 0202 434116

Products for Aromatherapy

Body and Soul,
Sarnett House,
Repton Drive,
Gidea Park,
Essex RM2 5LP
Tel: 0708 20289

Anita Phillips, who runs Body and Soul, sells a range of cosmetics and essential oils. She also conducts seminars on subjects such as Practical Aromatherapy.

There are lotions and creams for people prone to such things as eczema or psoriasis. There is also an anti-stress skin care range. The prices of essential oils vary from about £2 to £10 for 10 ml. The prices of Rose, Neroli and Jasmine Absolute will be given at the time of the enquiry. Items such as pottery oil burners can also be purchased.

Shirley Price Aromatherapy,
80 Castle Street,
Hinckley,
Leics. LE10 1DD
Supply essential oils by mail order, also mixes for particular purposes.

Suppliers of Medicinal Herbs and Prepared Herbal Remedies

Neal's Yard Apothecary,
2 Neal's Yard,
Covent Garden,
London WC2
Supply dried herbs from the shop or by mail order, also other herbs and products.

Cathay of Bournemouth Ltd.,
Hampshire House,
Bourne Avenue,
Bournemouth BH2 6DW
Tel: 0202 417452
Supply herbal remedies, herbal preparations for skin and hair care, and a wide range of dried herbs.

G. Baldwin and Co.,
173 Walworth Road,
London SE17 1RW
Tel: 01 703 5550
Supply dried herbs, essential oils and other herbal preparations, also books.

D. Napier and Sons Herbalists,
17 and 18 Bristo Place,
Edinburgh EH1 IHA
Tel: 031-225-5542
Supply a wide range of culinary and medicinal herbs.

Rayner and Pennycook,
PO Box 146,
Weybridge,
Surrey KT13 0SQ
Supply some herbs and oils for use in your own remedies and preparations. Also supply many remedies and products of their own.

The following companies usually sell their products through chemists and health shops. However, if you have difficulty obtaining a product, or require further information, contact the publicity/information officer at the relevant company:

Heath and Heather,
Beaver House,
York Close,
Byfleet,
Surrey.

A. Nelson & Co Ltd,
5 Endeavour Way,
London SW19 9UH

G.R. Lane Health Products Ltd,
Sisson Road,
Gloucester GL1 3QB

Potter's Herbal Supplies Ltd,
Leyland Mill Lane,
Wigan,
Lancs. WN1 25B

Weleda (UK) Ltd,
Heanor Road,
Ilkeston,
Derbyshire DE7 8DR

Hofels Pure Plant Supplements,
Stowmarket Road,
Woolpit,
Bury St. Edmunds,
Suffolk

Herbal Laboratories,
Copse Road,
Fleetwood,
Lancashire FY7 7PF

E.G. Marketing Ltd,
Swains Park Industrial Estate,
Park Road,
Overseal,
Burton-on-Trent,
Staffs DE12 6JT

Counsellor,
The Three Pines,
Church Road,
Penn,
Bucks. HP10 8EG

Organisations and Societies

The Herb Society,
77 Great Peter Street,
London SW1
Tel: 01-222-3634

The aim of the society is to collect and disseminate information about herbs. A quarterly publication, *The Herbal Review*, is sent to members who can also buy the society's books and leaflets at a discount. There are also some occasional lectures and seminars.

The Hardy Plant Society,
General Secretary,
Mrs. J. Sambrook,
Garden Cottage,
214 Ruxley Lane,
West Ewell,
Surrey KT17 9EU

This society does not supply plants. It produces a directory called

The Plant Finder which lists 40,000 plants with details of where to find them. It is a society for plant enthusiasts.

There is also a bulletin called *The Hardy Plant*. Slides are available from a central collection to members wishing to give lectures.

National Institute of Medical Herbalists,
41 Hatherley Road,
Winchester,
Hants.

The School of Herbal Medicine,
148 Forest Road,
Tunbridge Wells,
Kent TN2 5EY

Drinks

Norfolk Punch

This is a traditional non-alcoholic drink based on a medieval recipe. If you cannot obtain it from a health shop or large off-licence, contact:

Original Norfolk Punch,
Welle Manor Hall,
Upwell,
Norfolk PE14 9AB

The drink contains a wide range of herbs: fennel, alchoof, sweet basil, bay, angelica, camomile, caraway, dandelion, daisy, dock, liquorice, poppy, privet, cinnamon, ginger, clove, rosemary, sorrel, blackcurrant, hops, elderberry, peppermint, balm, vervain, thyme, rosewater, comfrey, ground ivy, feverfew and samphire.

The name Welle Manor Farm comes from a nearby natural spring which provides good, fresh water despite sources of salty water nearby. The water from the spring has traces of silenium, believed by some to be an aid to longevity. In addition to Norfolk Punch various associated products can also be purchased.

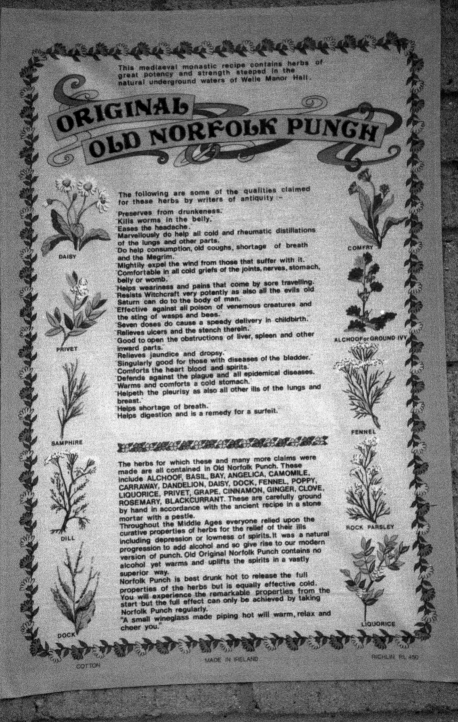

This mediaeval monastic recipe contains herbs of great potency and strength steeped in the natural underground waters of Welle Manor Hall.

ORIGINAL OLD NORFOLK PUNCH

The following are some of the qualities claimed for these herbs by writers of antiquity :—

Preserves from drunkeness.
Kills worms in the belly.
Eases the headache.
Marvellously do help all cold and rheumatic distillations of the lungs and other parts.
Do help consumption, old coughs, shortage of breath and the Megrim.
Mightily expel the wind from those that suffer with it.
Comfortable in all cold griefs of the joints, nerves, stomach, belly or womb.
Helps weariness and pains that come by sore travelling.
Resists Witchcraft very potently as also all the evils old Saturn can do to the body of man.
Effective against all poison of venemous creatures and the sting of wasps and bees.
Seven doses do cause a speedy delivery in childbirth.
Relieves ulcers and the stench therein.
Good to open the obstructions of liver, spleen and other inward parts.
Relieves jaundice and dropsy.
Singularly good for those with diseases of the bladder.
Comforts the heart blood and spirits.
Defends against the plague and all epidemical diseases.
Warms and comforts a cold stomach.
Helpeth the pleurisy as also all other ills of the lungs and breast.
Helps shortage of breath.
Helps digestion and is a remedy for a surfeit.

The herbs for which these and many more claims were made are all contained in Old Norfolk Punch. These include ALCHOOF, BASIL, BAY, ANGELICA, CAMOMILE, CARRAWAY, DANDELION, DAISY, DOCK, FENNEL, POPPY, LIQUORICE, PRIVET, GRAPE, CINNAMON, GINGER, CLOVE, ROSEMARY, BLACKCURRANT. These are carefully ground by hand in accordance with the ancient recipe in a stone mortar with a pestle.
Throughout the Middle Ages everyone relied upon the curative properties of herbs for the relief of their ills including depression or lowness of spirits. It was a natural progression to add alcohol and so give rise to our modern version of punch. Old Original Norfolk Punch contains no alcohol yet warms and uplifts the spirits in a vastly superior way.
Norfolk Punch is best drunk hot to release the full properties of the herbs but is equally effective cold. You will experience the remarkable properties from the start but the full effect can only be achieved by taking Norfolk Punch regularly.
"A small wineglass made piping hot will warm, relax and cheer you."

DAISY
PRIVET
SAMPHIRE
DILL
DOCK
COMFRY
ALCHOOF or GROUND IVY
FENNEL
ROCK PARSLEY
LIQUORICE

COTTON   MADE IN IRELAND   RICHLIN RL 450

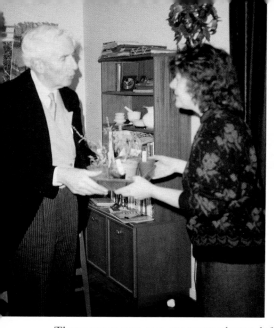

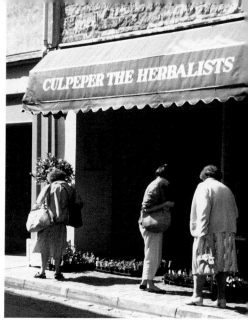

Three ways you can get your plants: *left*, personal delivery (Sir Peter Wells); *right*, from a shop (Culpeper); *bottom*, at a fair (display by John Chambers at 'game' fair).

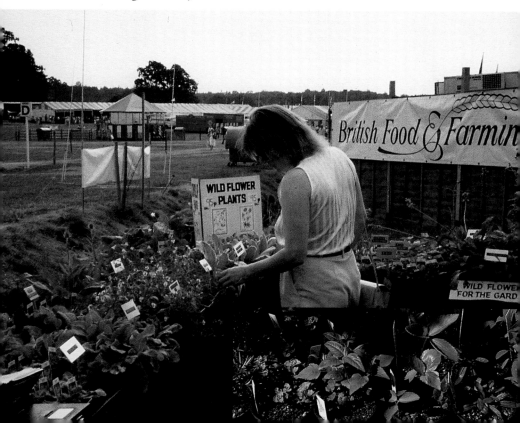

Sloe Gin

This is a drink that can be made at home or purchased.

Hawker's Sloe Gin has long been established as an English liqueur. The firm was founded by William Henry Hawker (1782-1862) and the original recipe remains a secret. Although most people drink Sloe Gin neat, Hawker's recommend several variations, such as:

Sloe Gin Fizz

One measure Hawker's Sloe
  Gin
Half measure lemon squash

One teaspoon castor sugar
One white of egg

Top up with soda water, shake well, and serve with ice, cherry and lemon.

Cosmetics and Toiletries

> Floral Fragrances Ltd,
> Porter's Vaults,
> Chapel Street,
> Thirsk,
> North Yorkshire Y07 1LU

This company produces luxury products, items for the perfume connoisseur. Their soaps, produced from English rose oil, are part of a *limited edition!* They come in an elegant box complete with a history of rose oil, each set costing about £150. They are part of Floral Fragrance's beautiful and growing selection of boudoir products.

For less expensive tastes, branches of the Body Shop provide an interesting range of herbal products, including such things as Aromatherapy Oils and Aromatherapy Massage Lotion.

Other manufacturers, such as Max Factor, also offer herbal products. Their Blasé range of products is produced with herbs and flowers renowned for their invigorating qualities — users should look and feel good!

Herbal toiletries which have not been tested on animals can be obtained by mail order from:

BUAV,
16a Crane Grove,
London N7 8LB

And firms such as Yardley maintain a long tradition of herbal products particularly from roses and lavender.
To visit:
Per Fumum Exhibition of Perfumery,
Cotswold Perfumery,
Bourton-on-the-Water,
Gloucestershire.
Tel: 0451 20698

More places to visit are listed at the end of Chapter 7.

Special Offers

The popularity of herbs has encouraged various companies to use them as a basis for special offers. Ruddles Brewery, Oakham, found an ingenious purpose for their used beer bottles. Customers could apply for sets of corks and labels to turn them into sets of herb containers.

Danbury Mint (Chessington, Surrey) produce a set of Flower Fairies Spice Jars featuring characters such as the Chive Fairy, the Sweet Marjoram Fairy, and the Tarragon Fairy, all in the tradition of Cicely Mary Barker.

Publicity Officer,
The Schwartz Herb & Spice Centre,
Dormer Road,
Thame,
Oxon. OX9 3SI.

As part of the promotion of their products, Schwartz provide information, charts, and small samples of new items.

Country Fairs and Shows

Herbs and related products are often featured in the crafts section of County Shows and similar events such as the annual Game Fair. Companies like John Chambers participate in some of these, providing an opportunity to examine items usually only encountered in a catalogue.

Information

In addition to the sources of information already listed, most of the major non-fiction publishers include a herb book for the general reader in their list. There are also certain specialist publishers who provide books for those looking in more detail at particular aspects of herbs or natural remedies. Some of these publishers are listed below.

Publishers do not supply books direct to customers but their publicity officer will send a catalogue and you can then order through a bookshop.

Blandford Press,
Artillery House,
Artillery Row,
London SW1P 1RT

C.W. Daniel & Co Ltd,
1 Church Path,
Saffron Walden,
Essex CB10 1 JP

David and Charles,
Brunei House,
Newton Abbot,
Devon TQ12 4PU

Ebury Press,
Colquhoun House,
27-37 Broadwick Street,
London W1V 1FR

Element Books,
Longmead,
Shaftesbury, Dorset, SP7 8PL

Thorsons Ltd,
Denington Estate,
Wellingborough,
Northants. NN8 2RQ

Tynron Press
Thornhill
Dumfriesshire DG3 4LD
Scotland

Selling Your Surplus Herbs and Herb Products

Plants

Some plants grown from seed — marjoram, for example — produce great numbers of seedlings. There will probably be far more than you need, and the surplus could be sold. This can sometimes be organised at local events, and some privately-owned shops will take produce in small amounts if the quality is reliable.

The plants will need to be in containers, and this must be considered in any price you ask. You may have some spare plastic pots, otherwise there are soft plastic containers which can be bought packed flat — these come at a very reasonable price.

Cards

Those decorated with real pressed flowers and leaves make a pleasant change if the price is reasonable. If you intend to make your own cards, rather than buy blanks, (available from some art suppliers and used by schools and playgroups) consider the possible greetings. If you are good at calligraphy, the design of any greetings should not be a problem. Otherwise, many commercially produced cards are now sold blank, and you could do the same.

The flowers and leaves must be thoroughly pressed and dried, and firmly stuck to the card. It is best to display the cards in cellophane packets if possible — as they are examined by customers and shuffled about, the design on uncovered cards may become loosened or damaged.

Before selecting your herbs, check their meanings and associations. Not all flowers send kind or happy messages!

Herb-scented candles

These can take some time to make and moreover, ornamental candles can be quite expensive, so you may find quite a few customers if you take pleasure in a hobby with a small return. It is important to sample the candles to check that the wicks are good and work well.

Pot Pourri

The price of the mixture will vary considerably according to the range of ingredients. The outlet you find will also influence the price range. Containers must also be considered. The mixture could just be sold in transparent bags, or sachets, baskets and boxes could be used and form part of the design.

Herb-flavoured preserves

Flavours such as minted apple jelly, rose hip jelly, blackcurrant cheese or quince marmalade are always popular, particularly if the presentation is attractive and original. This is the type of thing that people enjoy seeing at summer fairs.

Herb butter is also popular but needs to be displayed in the shade, or in a cool-bag. It is simple to make if you have some good, fresh herbs and unsalted butter. Cream the butter until fluffy, then add the herbs to taste. Press into shape or use butter pats.

Herb plants in bowls or bottles

Many smaller herbs can be used in bowl and bottle gardens. When you are planning the arrangement, consider the lid or stopper that will be used, if necessary. You will need to keep these for some time before they are ready and maturing.

You can create a traditional herb-garden on a small scale using plants such as miniature roses, thyme, pennyroyal, and so on.

Dried herbs

These could be sold in bunches or containers but quite a large surplus is required before you can do this. Herbs shrink as they dry, and if you rub them down for containers, you may be surprised at the amount you require.

Gifts

The above items make attractive gifts, as well as being suitable for sale. However, there are some home-made products that may only be suitable for a particular purpose — for example, cosmetics and simple remedies could be a problem if sold. You will not know of any allergies or problems that particular purchasers may suffer from. But if you make such things for your friends, you can discuss them fully first.

A Reposé of Herbs

A refreshing period of calm at the end of the evening provides time to reflect on the day's events or to make plans for tomorrow. Unwinding successfully usually requires a comfortable setting: a favourite chair, loose clothes, no interruptions. Quite a few herbs are noted for their relaxing properties — and they work best in harmonious surroundings. For some people, certain colours are effective. For others, music or particular images are more potent. You may have a clear idea of these, or you may be surprised at the effect a few changes can make.

The prospect of deep, peaceful sleep puts you in a better frame of mind during the day. Freedom from the worry of sleeplessness, and confidence that the night will restore lost energies, can give new life to daytime activities. Some sleepless nights are a natural part of most people's sleep patterns but regular sleepless nights are a problem.

If you want to improve your sleep pattern, or establish a new one, herbs can provide a range of gentle, natural routes to restful sleep. Many act as aids to a pleasant, relaxing evening.

Before making any changes in your routine, you will need to feel sure that sleeplessness is not caused by any particular physical difficulties or mental stress. If there is an underlying cause, it will need attention, though a period of relaxation would undoubtedly still be helpful.

The remedies and recipes set out below cover quite a wide range of flavours and fragrances. Try to find ones that you particularly enjoy as this will contribute to their effect.

Drinks

Relaxing tisanes and infusions

The following herbs are all suitable for this purpose: camomile flowers, lime blossom, red clover flowers, hop flowers, rosemary leaves, lemon verbena leaves, skullcap leaves and flowers, and hyssop leaves and flowers.

Prepare a tisane if you simply want a warm relaxing drink at the end of the evening. If you require something stronger, prepare an amount equal to several infusions (see page 88) and drink them at intervals during the evening.

As these drinks are to be part of a relaxing evening, it is best to have your herbs and any other ingredients prepared and ready as required.

If you are using freshly-picked herbs, keep them away from dust and cooking smells. Also, check the amount. Quite large quantities are needed when fresh herbs are used.

If you are using dried herbs, make sure that they are in the form required. If, for example, you want to use camomile flowers but have dried whole plants, remove the flower heads and put them in a suitable container.

If you are using roots or woody stems, make sure these are broken into pieces. And if you are using some of the tougher seeds, bruise them first.

In some cases, you might want to make your own tea bags. Muslin can be used for this, and you will know how much is required for each bag by trial and error.

As you are making a tisane or infusion for a purpose, not simply as a refreshing drink, it is important that none of the properties of the herb are lost. If you intend to boil the herb in a saucepan, use one with a lid, or some of the oils may evaporate. Otherwise, use an infuser or a suitable teapot. In winter, when you may want more hot drinks during the night, make an amount equal to several infusions, and keep the liquid in a thermos.

In summer, you may prefer a cold drink at the end of the evening. In this case, you can either make the amount you require in the usual way and cool it, or you can prepare a cold infusion.

Cold infusion

For use at night, prepare this at midday or mid-morning as it needs to stand. Use the same proportions as for one or more standard infusions, but use cold water or cold milk. Put the mixture into a covered glass or china container until the evening, then strain.

Tinctures with alcohol

In order not to conflict with the flavour of the herb, an alcoholic drink such as vodka or dry white wine is best. Tinctures are much stronger than infusions or decoctions, so only small amounts are required. They can be added to water or to alcohol. For example, if you have made your tincture with dry white wine, you can add a few drops of it to a glass of dry white wine. This will provide a pleasant, herb-flavoured bedtime drink.

The following herbs can all be used for sleep-inducing tinctures: Californian poppy (leaves and flowers), passion flower (leaves), valerian (roots), camomile (flowers), lime blossom (flowers) and red clover (flowers).

Up to about 4 ml can be added to an evening drink. Take one or two drinks during the evening if required.

Items required

¼ lb dried herbs
1 pint alcoholic drink
  (such as vodka or
  dry white wine)

¾ lb fresh herbs —
  rubbed or chopped
large wine bottle
plastic funnel

Preparation

1. Mix herbs and alcohol.
2. Pour through funnel into bottle.
3. Keep for 10-14 days, shaking at least daily.
4. Strain into a dark bottle for storage.

Relaxation

You may want to combine your evening use of herbs with a relaxation technique. Some people find that strenuous exercise is followed by a feeling of peace and calm. Others look for a gentler route.

If you have attended relaxation classes (either for general purposes, or perhaps during pregnancy) you may have tried a widely-used test which can reveal areas of tension and at the same time bring relaxation. It follows a very simple pattern and requires no equipment or special instruments.

First, make sure that you are comfortable, either sitting or lying down. Wear no shoes.

Then, starting with your toes, tighten the muscles for a few seconds, release, and rest. Next, tighten your calf muscles, hold, and release. Bring your knees up as far as possible, hold, and release. Gradually, move up your body, tightening and releasing your muscles, until you reach your face. Then, screw up your eyes, release and relax . . . wrinkle your nose, release and relax . . . smile as wide as possible, then pout. Try to wiggle your ears.

At the end of your exercises, rest. After a few minutes, prepare your chosen herbal drink. If possible, have an activity ready that will be interesting but not demanding: sorting last year's holiday photos, looking through a new recipe book, writing a letter to an old friend, stroking the cat, reading a book for armchair sportsmen, or making plans you might never use for new colour schemes throughout your home.

Alongside physical exercises, there are also various written exercises that can be helpful if you feel that anxiety or stress may be preventing relaxation. If you have had a bad day, try writing down the ten most annoying things that happened. Spend a little time sorting them in order — worst first, more bearable, last. Then think back to a good day. Write down, in order, the ten things that made it work well. Compare your lists to see if contrasts suggest any changes you could make. Then read your list for the good day again.

During times of stress and anxiety, there are various herbs likely to be helpful:

Lady's slipper (*Cypripedium pubescens*) — take a decoction of the roots;

Vervain (*Verbena officinalis*) — take an infusion of the aerial parts;

Wild oats (*Avena sativa*) — take an infusion of the whole plant;

Valerian (*Valeriana officinalis*) — take a decoction of the roots;

Wood betony (*Stachys betonica*) — take an infusion of the aerial parts;

St. John's Wort (*Hypericum perforatum*) — take an infusion of the aerial parts.

Other plants, such as pasque flower (*Anemone pulsatilla*) and crampbark (*Viburnam opulus*) can be used with the guidance of a qualified herbalist.

Fragrant Baths

It is possible to prepare a relaxing bath using an infusion or decoction of any of the herbs mentioned above. Just prepare the ingredients in the usual way, strain, and add to the bath. However, for fragrance another herb must be added.

There are also some herbs which can be used for fragrance *and* relaxation. These include: lavender (*Lavandula officinalis*), rosemary (*Rosemarinus officinalis*), lemon balm (*Melissa officinalis*), sweet violet flowers (*Viola odorata*).

At times when you feel that an invigorating bath might be suitable, perhaps as a prelude to relaxing activities, add about ¼ pint of herb vinegar to your bath. Choose a vinegar flavoured by a herb with appropriate properties.

Essential oils provide a simple way to prepare a fragrant bath. Add about 5 or 6 drops of the chosen oil to a warm, but not hot, bath. (If you have no time for a bath, sprinkle a few drops of oil on a tissue, and inhale now and then as you continue your activities.)

The following essential oils are all suitable for relaxing baths: basil, camomile, clary sage, geranium, lavender, marjoram, orange blossom, rosemary, sage, lemon, mandarin, cedarwood or ylang-ylang.

Diet

Regular, balanced meals contribute towards a healthy, relaxed lifestyle. You may eat meat or you may be a vegetarian. You may follow a particular diet, perhaps macrobiotic or high-fibre, or you may enjoy food from a certain country or region. Some diets are healthier than others — but whatever your preferences, it is always worthwhile to check certain features.

In developed countries, many foods with a high sugar or fat content have flooded the market. Additives have been used in processing, and valuable parts of some foods are no longer included in the finished product. As well as these considerations, each person has individual needs, and these vary according to time of life.

Too much sugar can contribute to tiredness and depression by causing changing blood sugar levels. Try to keep your sugar intake as low as possible. If you find you need to use an artificial sweetener, check several types before making a choice, and note the substances used.

Animal products provide necessary protein but in excess they are thought to contribute to such problems as hypertension. This is more likely to be a problem with red meats than with poultry, game or offal which are lower in fat, and which also offer more nutrients.

Some people — thought to be about 3 to 15 in every 10,000 but very likely more — react to additives. In Britain, there are four main categories: preservatives, antioxidants, emulsifiers and stabilisers, and colours. Each additive has a number, and if recognised by the EEC, it also has an 'E' by the number.

Certain additives are known to cause more reaction than others. These include Tatrazine (E102), Caramel (E150), Sunset Yellow (E110), and Benzoic Acid (E210). These, and any others included in a product, are listed on the packaging.

If you would like more information about additives, you can obtain a booklet called 'Food Additives' from:

> Ministry of Agriculture Fisheries and Food,
> Publications Unit,
> Lion House,
> Willowburn Trading Estate,
> Alnwick,
> Northumberland NE66 2PF.

In addition to noting these features of your diet, some attention to the use of herbs can improve the dishes prepared, aid digestion, and provide various vitamins, minerals and trace elements which may not be present in the main ingredients.

Herbs to aid digestion

Some herbs traditionally used as accompaniments to particular foods will aid digestion while they provide an appropriate flavour. Horseradish, mint, rosemary and garlic are included in this group.

Various other herbs, often with mild flavours, have proved popular in food for invalids. Marjoram is suitable for this use — it blends well with light meat dishes and vegetables.

Watercress added to salad will aid digestion, and a meal can end with a dessert flavoured by such things as ginger, coriander or cardamon — all remedies for indigestion.

Herbs and vitamins

Vitamin C and the B group of vitamins are important aids to relaxation. They help the body cope with physical and mental stress. In addition to providing some of these vitamins, herbs can also enhance food and drink prepared to aid vitamin intake.

Milk and fruit drinks are a pleasant source of some of these vitamins. Variety, and additional benefits, can be provided by herbs.

Cool summer drinks

Apple juice with cinnamon

A change from plain apple juice — use a liquid spice if you want to avoid the sediment left by dried cinnamon.

Pomegranate juice with grenadine

Juice from fresh pomegranates has a distinctive taste and provides a change from the more usual juices. The fruit also looks very attractive while you are keeping it. Probably because of the large number of seeds they contain, pomegranates are regarded as a symbol of fertility in many areas. Take care with the preparation as the juice contains a dye.

Items required

Several pomegranates
A few drops of grenadine
Mineral water
(A measure of vodka if an alcoholic drink is preferred)

Preparation

1. Scoop out the seeds and press gently to extract the juice. Take care not to crush too many seeds or you will spoil the taste.
2. Add a few drops of grenadine.
3. Add a measure of vodka if required.
4. Top up with mineral water.

Grapefruit juice with mint

Pour a carton of grapefruit juice into a china or glass container. Add several chopped sprigs of mint and stand for a few hours. Strain before serving.

Spiced, iced coffee

This can be made most easily using a liquid coffee such as 'Camp'. Try a coffee substitute such as dandelion root if you would like to experiment. Make the coffee to the usual strength per person but use only a small amount of water. Add liquid spices to taste. Add the milk, and stand in the fridge. Serve in glasses with ice cubes.

Warm winter drinks

Marmite with mixed herbs

Drinks such as Marmite and Bovril are good for the B group of vitamins. The taste can be varied by adding a few drops of liquid mixed herbs.

Cider Cup

Items required

Carton of apple juice	4 cloves
1 pint of cider	2 teaspoons dark brown sugar
1 cinnamon stick	Apple slices

Preparation

1. Heat all the ingredients gently for a few minutes. Keep the temperature well below boiling point.
2. Strain the liquid into a suitable container.
3. Serve garnished with apple slices.

Spiced Milk

Items required

1 pint milk	1 teaspoon ground ginger
1 measure ginger wine	1 teaspoon dark brown sugar

Preparation

1. Heat the milk gently. Do not bring to the boil.
2. Add the other ingredients and continue heating below boiling point.
3. Serve in mugs or heatproof glasses.

Vitamins from edible seaweeds

Edible seaweeds such as laver, dulse and carragheen are popular for invalids as they are nourishing and easily digested. For anyone who enjoys the taste, they are a good source of vitamins A, B, C, D and K. They are also one of the few plant sources of B12. If you have difficulty obtaining seaweeds locally, try:

Clearspring,
196 Old Street,
London EC1.
They supply from the shop or through mail order.

Relaxing Fragrances from Pot-Pourri

A light fresh fragrance

Lemon balm (*Melissa officinalis*)
Camomile (*Matricaria chamomilla*)
Lemon verbena (*Lippia citriodora*)
Lemon eucalyptus (*Eucalyptus citriodora*)
Clary sage (*Salvia sclarea*)

Prepare in the usual way. As time passes, the fragrance can be freshened with lemon or melissa oil.

A soft summer fragrance

Sweet violet (*Viola odorata*)
Lavender (*Lavandula officinalis*)
Rose petals (select for fragrance)
Geranium (any scented variety)
Woodruff (*Asperula odorata*)

Prepare in the usual way. As time passes, the fragrance can be freshened with geranium or lavender oil.

Other Aids

Supplements

Ginseng

This is often taken as an antidote to stress. It is a good source of vitamins B1, B2, and B12. There are two main types: *Panax quinquefolia* (from North America) and *Panax ginseng* (from Asia).

It is one of the best-known tonics in the world, and is sold in many different grades. The best grades have at times been sold at prices higher than gold. If you decide to use it, check the area of origin and grade against the price.

If you find ginseng too expensive as a regular tonic, you could try ginseng tea.

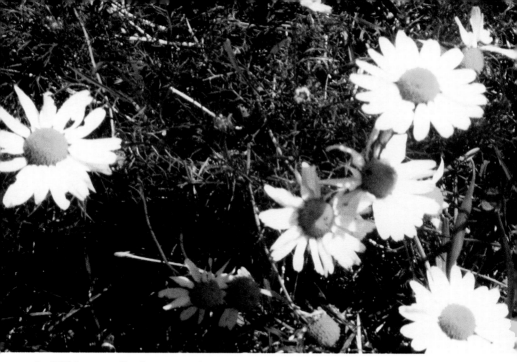

△ Wild camomile flowers make a refreshing tisane.

▽ Red clover can be used in a bedtime drink.

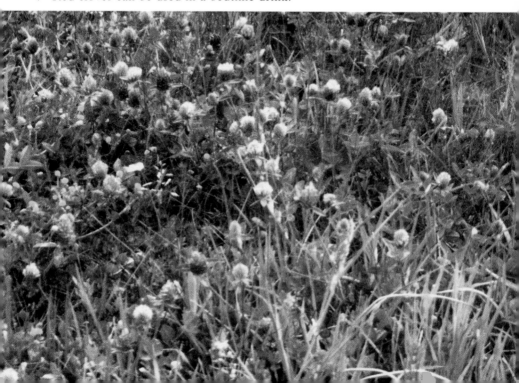

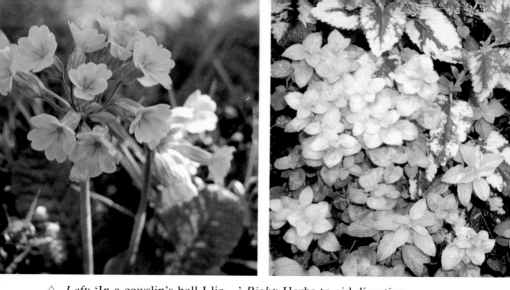

△ *Left*: 'In a cowslip's bell I lie ...' *Right*: Herbs to aid digestion — variegated mint and marjoram.

▽ Lemon balm for a fragrant and relaxing bath.

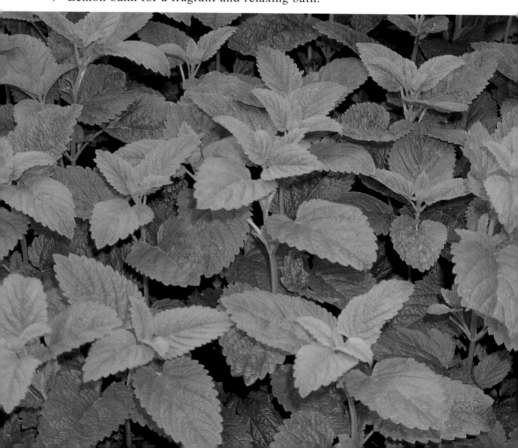

Evening Primrose Oil

Evening primrose oil (*Oenothera biennis*) is particularly effective as an antidote to stress caused by premenstrual syndrome (PMS). It is also a good general tonic, helpful for such things as brittle nails and, possibly, hyperactivity in children.

The special properties of the plant have been recognised for many years, especially by the North American Indians. The oil provides fatty acids, particularly gamma-linolenic acid in a form acceptable to the body.

Royal Jelly

This acts as a general tonic, particularly by providing a natural source of B vitamins, and vitamins C and F. Its effect is thought to depend largely on pantothenic acid which may vary considerably in strength. If you decide to use royal jelly, try various sources and select the one which seems most potent.

The Bach Flower Remedies

The Bach flower remedies are intended for use at home, and it is advised that you should start by choosing the two remedies most likely to help. Others can then be added as time passes. With this in mind, if you are looking for an aid in dealing with general physical and mental stress, you might choose a remedy such as 'olive', or select a more specific remedy such as 'white chestnut' for worrying thoughts, or 'agrimony' for hidden worry.

Air Ionizers

Positive ions produced by such things as central heating and smoking can cause feelings of depression. An ionizer helps to counteract this tendency.

Herb-scented Pillows

Any dried, fragrant, relaxing herb can be used to stuff pillows.

Hops have proved popular because they are sleep inducing *and* produce a soft pillow. Other sleep-inducing herbs could be used — if they are not soft when dried they can be mixed with feathers or foam.

For those people who find even hops uncomfortable, select a suitable pillow and sprinkle it with a few drops of an appropriate oil, such as orange blossom, lemon, mandarin or lavender.

Some Reflections on Herbs

During your relaxing evening, you could give some thought to herbs and their special properties. By using them, you have joined a long tradition. Archaeologists tell us that their value was probably recognised by Neanderthal man as he struggled to make his life more bearable. Poppy and hollyhock were amongst the earliest herbs in use, and they remain in use today.

References to herbs show how the meaning of the word has changed. In the Old Testament, 'herb' embraces a wide range of plants, perhaps all of them: 'Even as the green herb have I given you all things'.

During the classic eras of the knot garden and parterre, references to herbs occurred in many contexts:

Go, and catch a falling star,
Get with child a mandrake root,
Tell me, where all past years are,
Or who cleft the Devil's foot.

John Donne

And who gave thee this jolly red nose?
Nutmeg and ginger, cinnamon and cloves . . .

Frances Beaumont and John Fletcher

Down with the Rosemary and so
Down with the Bayes and Mistletoe:
Down with the Holly, Ivy, all,
Wherewith ye drest the Christmas Hall;
That so the superstitious find
Not one least branch there left behind . . .

Robert Herrick

Some of our most enduring images of herbs come from this period:

The rose by any other name would smell as sweet.

Romeo and Juliet, Shakespeare.

Where the bee sucks, there suck I,
In a cowslip's bell I lie . . .

The Tempest, Shakespeare

Out of this nettle, danger, we pluck this flower, safety.

King Henry IV Part I, Shakespeare

The current revival of interest in herbs is producing a new and changing vocabulary. Our herbs are more clearly defined. They are usually plants with particular culinary, medicinal or fragrant properties. We will leave future generations expressions such as 'green revolution', 'natural energy', 'holistic medicine', and 'organic farming'. To give these terms real meaning, the period that coined them should also pass on a herb-friendly environment that has been treated with care and respect.

EVERGREEN FOLIAGE

NAME	ANNUAL BIENNIAL PERENNIAL	HEIGHT	SPREAD	SUN/SHADE	FLOWER COLOUR
Aloe (*Aloe vera*)	PERENNIAL	VARIES GREATLY UP TO ABOUT 2 METRES IN BRITAIN	ABOUT 1 METRE	SUN/SHADE	CREAMY YELLOW
Juniper (*Juniperus communis*)	PERENNIAL	UP TO ABOUT 7 METRES	ABOUT 5 METRES	SUN/SOME SHADE	YELLOW FLOWERS/ BLUE BERRIES
Lavender (*Lavandula officinalis*)	PERENNIAL	75 CMS	60 CMS	SUN/SOME SHADE	BLUE/ PURPLE
Lemon balm (*Melissa officinalis*)	PERENNIAL	50 CMS	AS ALLOWED TO SPREAD	SUN/SOME SHADE	WHITE/ YELLOW
Parsley (*Petroselinum crispum*)	ANNUAL OR BIENNIAL	30 CMS	20 CMS	SUN/SHADE	CREAM/ WHITE

EVERGREEN FOLIAGE

NAME	ANNUAL BIENNIAL PERENNIAL	HEIGHT	SPREAD	SUN/SHADE	FLOWER COLOUR
Periwinkle (*Vinca major*)	PERENNIAL	40 CMS	AS ALLOWED TO SPREAD	SUN/ SHADE	MAUVE
Rosemary (*Rosmarinus officinalis*)	PERENNIAL	1 METRE	1.5 METRES	SUN	BLUE
Rue (*Ruta graveolens*)	PERENNIAL	60 CMS	50 CMS	SUN/A LITTLE SHADE	YELLOW
Sage (*Salvia officinalis*)	PERENNIAL	60 CMS	60 CMS	SUN/ A LITTLE SHADE	MAUVE
Sweet bay (*Laurus nobilis*)	PERENNIAL	20-30 FEET	AS ALLOWED TO SPREAD		CREAM FLOWERS PURPLE BERRIES

EVERGREEN FOLIAGE

NAME	ANNUAL BIENNIAL PERENNIAL	HEIGHT	SPREAD	SUN/SHADE	FLOWER COLOUR
Thyme (*Thymus vulgaris*)	PERENNIAL	10-15 CMS	AS ALLOWED TO SPREAD	SUN	PALE LILAC
Winter savory (*Satureja montana*)	PERENNIAL	30 CMS	30 CMS	SUN	PALE PINK
Vervain (*Verbena officinalis*)	PERENNIAL	UP TO ABOUT 75 CMS	AS ALLOWED TO SPREAD	SUN	LILAC
Wormwood (*Artimisia absinthum*)	PERENNIAL	1 METRE	30-40 CMS	SUN/SHADE	GREEN/ YELLOW

DARK GREEN FOLIAGE

NAME	ANNUAL BIENNIAL PERENNIAL	HEIGHT	SPREAD	SUN/SHADE	FLOWER COLOUR
Angelica (*Angelica archangelica*)	BIENNIAL/ OCCASIONAL PERENNIAL	2 METRES	1 METRE	SHADE	YELLOW
Bergamot (*Monarda didyma*)	PERENNIAL	60 CMS	30 CMS	SUN/SOME SHADE	RED
Borage (*Borago officinalis*)	ANNUAL	60 CMS	30 CMS	SUN	BLUE/PINK/ WHITE
Bugle (*Ajuga reptans*)	PERENNIAL	20 CMS	30 CMS	SUN/SHADE	BLUE
Chives (*Allium schoenoprasum*)	PERENNIAL	20 CMS	AS ALLOWED TO SPREAD	SUN/SHADE	PINK/ PURPLE

DARK GREEN FOLIAGE

NAME	ANNUAL BIENNIAL PERENNIAL	HEIGHT	SPREAD	SUN/SHADE	FLOWER COLOUR
Coriander (*Coriandum sativum*)	ANNUAL	50 CMS	30 CMS	SUN	PINK
Dill (*Anethum graveolens*)	ANNUAL	75 CMS	60 CMS	SUN	YELLOW
Elecampagne (*Inula helenium*)	PERENNIAL	1-1.5 METRES	1 METRE	SUN	YELLOW
French Tarragon (*Artemisia dracunculus*)	PERENNIAL	80 CMS	40 CMS	SUN	WHITE
Hyssop (*Hysoppus officinalis*)	PERENNIAL	60 CMS	20 CMS	SUN	BLUE/PINK/ WHITE
Lily-of-the-valley (*Convallaria majolis*)	PERENNIAL	25 CMS	AS ALLOWED TO SPREAD	SUN/SHADE	WHITE

DARK GREEN FOLIAGE

NAME	ANNUAL BIENNIAL PERENNIAL	HEIGHT	SPREAD	SUN/SHADE	FLOWER COLOUR
Lovage (*Levisticum officinalis*)	PERENNIAL	2 METRES	1 METRE	SUN/SHADE	YELLOW
Mint (*Mentha piperita*)	PERENNIAL	60 CMS	AS ALLOWED TO SPREAD	SUN/SHADE	MAUVE
Saffron crocus (*Crocus sativus*)	PERENNIAL	30 CMS	15 CMS	SUN	MAUVE
Sweet marjoram (*Origanum majorana*)	PERENNIAL	25 CMS	15 CMS	SUN	PINK
Sweet violet (*Viola odorata*)	PERENNIAL	10 CMS	10 CMS	SUN/SHADE	VIOLET
Sweet woodruff (*Asperula odorata*)	PERENNIAL	25 CMS	AS ALLOWED TO SPREAD	SUN/SHADE	WHITE

DARK GREEN FOLIAGE

NAME	ANNUAL BIENNIAL PERENNIAL	HEIGHT	SPREAD	SUN/SHADE	FLOWER COLOUR
Tansy (*Tanacetum vulgare*)	PERENNIAL	1-5 METRES	1 METRE	SUN/SHADE	YELLOW
Tree Onion (*Allium cepa aggregatum*)	PERENNIAL	40 CMS	15 CMS	SUN	USUALLY ONLY GREENISH BUD SEEN
Watercress (*Nasturtium officinale*)	PERENNIAL	FLAT ON WATER OR WET LAND	ABOUT 60 CMS	SUN/SHADE	WHITE

MID-GREEN OR LIGHT GREEN FOLIAGE

NAME	ANNUAL BIENNIAL PERENNIAL	HEIGHT	SPREAD	SUN/SHADE	FLOWER COLOUR
Basil (*Ocimum basilicum*)	ANNUAL	35 CMS	15 CMS	SUN	CREAM
Calamint (*Calamintha officinalis*)	PERENNIAL	30 CMS	50 CMS	SUN	BLUE
Caraway (*Carum carvi*)	BIENNIAL	60 CMS	30 CMS	SUN	WHITE
Common Comfrey (*Symphytum officinalis*)	PERENNIAL	75 CMS	AS ALLOWED TO SPREAD	SUN/SHADE	BLUE & PINK
Corn Salad (*Valeriana locusta*)	ANNUAL	20 CMS	20 CMS	SUN/SHADE	MAUVE
Fennel (*Foeniculum vulgare*)	PERENNIAL	ABOUT 1 METRE	75 CMS	SUN	YELLOW

MID-GREEN OR LIGHT GREEN FOLIAGE

NAME	ANNUAL BIENNIAL PERENNIAL	HEIGHT	SPREAD	SUN/SHADE	FLOWER COLOUR
Honeysuckle (*Lonicera periclymenum*)	PERENNIAL	AS ALLOWED TO CLIMB	AS ALLOWED TO SPREAD	SUN/SHADE	YELLOW
Lady's mantle (*Alchemilla vulgaris*)	PERENNIAL	25 CMS	15 CMS	SUN/SHADE	YELLOW
Myrtle (*Myrtus communis*)	PERENNIAL	ABOUT 3 METRES	ABOUT 1.5 METRES	SUN/SHADE	WHITE
Nasturtium (*Tropaeolum majus*)	CAN BE GROWN AS ANNUAL OR PERENNIAL	CAN CLIMB TO ABOUT 3 METRES	AS ALLOWED TO SPREAD	SUN/SHADE	MAINLY YELLOW & ORANGE
Purslane (*Portulaca oleracea*)	ANNUAL	25 CMS	25 CMS	SUN	YELLOW

MID-GREEN OR LIGHT GREEN FOLIAGE

NAME	ANNUAL BIENNIAL PERENNIAL	HEIGHT	SPREAD	SUN/SHADE	FLOWER COLOUR
Roman Camomile (*Chamaemelum nobile*)	PERENNIAL	25 CMS	15 CMS	SUN/SHADE	WHITE
Russian Tarragon (*Artemisia dracunculoides*)	PERENNIAL	1 METRE	50 CMS	SUN	WHITE
Soapwort (*Saponaria officinalis*)	PERENNIAL	75 CMS	AS ALLOWED TO SPREAD	SUN/SHADE	PINK/WHITE
Wood Betony (*Stachys officinalis*)	PERENNIAL	75 CMS	25 CMS	SUN	PINK

GREY FOLIAGE

NAME	ANNUAL BIENNIAL PERENNIAL	HEIGHT	SPREAD	SUN/SHADE	FLOWER COLOUR
Clary (*Salvia scalarea*)	BIENNIAL OR PERENNIAL	80 CMS	25 CMS	SUN	BLUE
Costmary (*Chrysanthemum balsamita*)	PERENNIAL	1 METRE	50 CMS	SUN	YELLOW
Globe Artichoke (*Cynara scolymus*)	PERENNIAL	1.5 METRES	1 METRE	SUN	PURPLE
Horehound (white) (*Marrubium vulgare*)	PERENNIAL	50 CMS	AS ALLOWED TO SPREAD	SUN/SHADE	WHITE
Lavender (*Lavandula officinalis*)	PERENNIAL	75 CMS	60 CMS	SUN/SHADE	MAUVE
Mugwort (*Artemisia vulgaris*)	PERENNIAL	1-5 METRES	50 CMS	SUN/SHADE	YELLOW

GREY FOLIAGE

NAME	ANNUAL BIENNIAL PERENNIAL	HEIGHT	SPREAD	SUN/SHADE	FLOWER COLOUR
Opium poppy (*Papaver somniferum*)	ANNUAL	1 METRE	40 CMS	SUN/SHADE	PINK
Sage (*Salvia officinalis*)	PERENNIAL	60 CMS	60 CMS	SUN/A LITTLE SHADE	MAUVE
Wormwood (*Artimisia absinthum*)	PERENNIAL	1 METRE	50 CMS	SUN/SHADE	YELLOW